RUN THIS PLACE

by: Dane Rauschenberg

Martin,

Go get that BQ!

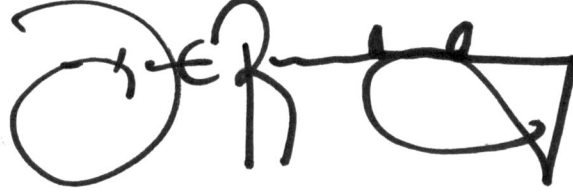

Run This Place
Copyright © 2018 by Dane Rauschenberg. All rights reserved.

No part of this publication may be reproduced, stored in a retrieval system or transmitted in any way by any means, electronic, mechanical, photocopy, recording or otherwise without the prior permission of the author except as provided by USA copyright law.

The opinions expressed by the author are not necessarily those of Trinity Press.

Cover design by Gregg Rauschenberg
Photos by Matt Jensen Photography
Front cover is Bonneville Salt Flats, Utah
Back Cover is Manchester, Maryland

Published by Trinity Press, Inc.
3190 Reps Miller Road
Suite 360
Norcross, GA 30071

Book Design copyright © 2018 by Trinity Press, Inc.

Published in the United States of America

ISBN: 978-0-9915940-1-6

Advance Praise for *Run This Place*

"I promised my aging self, 'I will not have a bucket list, I will not have a bucket list.' Doggone it, Dane, you've given me a bucket list!"

- Kathrine Switzer, first woman to officially run the Boston Marathon (1967)

"Just as we runners benefit from the knowledge of more experienced runners, so too can we learn about the unique aspects of races that lift us up. I know Dane and am confident his choice of races will get you motivated and energized to explore!"

- Bill Rodgers, four-time winner of Boston and NYC Marathons

The Warm Up

"What's your favorite marathon?"

Without a doubt this is one of the top three questions I am asked when at a book signing or speaking engagement. Given I am often signing a book about my first 100 marathons, this is not an unreasonable question.

That said, the answer is, more often than not: "I have no idea." Then I am asked for my top three or four favorites and I realize I still am at a loss. So many races have so many different values attached to them. I don't know where to begin with what is my favorite.

Why do I hedge so much on picking a favorite? First and foremost, I hope it is difficult for me to choose the best race I have ever run because I have yet to run that race. But after being posed the question so many times, I decided the optimal way to come up with a suitable solution was to sit down and think about all the marathons I had run. In doing so, while I have run more marathons than any other distance, other races popped into my mind. I thought of all the good times I had at events which were *not* the 26.2 distance. Some definitely stuck out over others.

As a voracious reader of all things running, I have always read articles which claim to have a list of "must-run" races. Time and time again, if there were ten races, seven of them would be the same. For the most part, I knew why that was the case.[1] I was also aware there were a plethora of races out there which never crack the national consciousness and lag behind in getting the attention they deserve. This is when it dawned on me I needed to make a list of *all* the running events I have enjoyed in order to share with those who were curious.

But what criteria should I use? Was it the race medal that stood out? Could it be the organization and the minutia behind the scenes? How about the attention to detail of the entire event top

---

[1] The thing about making a living in the running industry is you get to see behind the curtain. It's often not pretty. Like learning that "Race of the Month" picked by your venerable running mag got the nod because it paid for it. I know I am ruining things for you. Also, there is no Santa.

to bottom? Was it the challenge or lack thereof that attracted me? How much emphasis did I put on the beauty of the course itself? The answer is yes, all of that. In other words, like United States Supreme Court Justice Potter Stewart, who described his threshold test for obscenity in Jacobellis v. Ohio[2], "I know it when I see it." Or in this case, run it.

In pouring over these different characteristics I came to the conclusion that no matter what made my list, other people were still going to like races for their own special reasons. Runners have preferences which are as varied as the races we run. Some like trails and some like roads. Others like to run in big cities, while their buddies like to run in small towns. Some don't consider themselves a "real" runner until they have run an ultra, whereas their spouse has never run anything over a 5K and doesn't want to contemplate a step further. All I could do to meet the tastes of so many was to guide those who were curious to the races which stuck with me long after I crossed the finish line.

Some of the races in this book will be out of your present range of ability. Some you might have run already. But I have done everything in my power to find contests which offered something rather unique. I did my best to stay away from the "obvious" choices that I had seen time and time again in other similar lists. Nevertheless, some races are obvious for a good reason: you should run them.

What follows is a collection which not only tantalizes the senses but also titillates the mind. Moreover, every one of these races is one I have personally raced at least once. I have also taken into account the varying skill levels of runners who may be reading this book and have selected as many different types of races as possible without just adding fluff for fluff's sake. There will be some truly short and easy races and some extremely long and challenging races included within these pages. In addition, sometimes a race has multiple distances offered. Often I have singled out just one of those distances for a very good reason, so pay attention. There

---

[2] I went to law school.

will be a test.[3]

Understand this is not an exhaustive list of races. In fact, I have no doubt I could have doubled the sample size without decreasing the must-do-ness of the list. Regardless, there is nary a race on this vastly different assortment of distances which shouldn't add to your own personal to-do list.

Now all you have to do is go run them.

---

[3] You passed. Congratulations. This book is more valuable than a diploma from Trump University.

The Short-Timers: 5K and Their Ilk

Race: Harrisburg Mile

Typical Date: Third Wednesday in July

Distance: Mile

Location: Harrisburg, PA

Why You Should Run It:

To be upfront, I am going to use this first entry to say that you should really run any mile race you can. There is nothing more quintessentially American than the mile. Forget apple pie. Forget baseball. Unabashedly, while most of the world says Americans are too stubbornly stuck to the imperial system, we know the mile is where it is at. And you know what, so does everyone else. They are just afraid to admit it. No runner in any country talks about their kilometerage for the week. Or how Roger Bannister was the first person to break the four-minute 1.6 kilometer.[4] It's the mile, baby.

But the mile has fallen a bit on hard times as of late. It is rarely run in any international competition. In high school, the 1600 meter takes its place even though that is a maddening 9.3 meters short of a mile. Fortunately, there is a swelling of those fighting to bring back the mile. I count myself among them. So, while I am touting the Harrisburg Mile as a definite race you should run, I implore you to find as many of them as you can and race them. Do your job as an American![5]

Having said all of that, I chose the Harrisburg Mile for a variety of reasons. First, the race is not run in the morning as most races are; rather it starts at 6 p.m. As you will read throughout this book, I am not a morning person. How I even function on race morning is beyond me. Nothing will change this. For five years growing up, six days a week, I was up at 5 a.m. to deliver papers. I had early

---
[4] RIP.
[5] Cue fireworks and eagle release.

morning classes throughout college and law school. I clerked for a judge after I got my J.D. which required an early start. I worked in D.C. for four years which had me out the door to avoid traffic at 7:20 am. NONE of that made me a morning person. So a race that starts at 6 p.m.? Hells to the yes.

Second, unlike more than a few mile races which are more prestigious, this mile is run in an absolute straight line with no right angle turns, no curves, no nothing. You start, and I quote, "18 feet 11 inches southeast of the third lamp post northwest of Maclay Street" and end "on the northwest edge of the fire hydrant near Boas Street." Are you kidding me? How can you not love that!

Where do you run? On Front Street in Harrisburg, right along the Susquehanna River with a bank of homes you can't afford on your left and the river on your right. Line them up, fire the gun, and run.

Did I mention it is also on a Wednesday? I mean, seriously. The randomness of this race should have you signing up right now.

My Experience:

I ran this race after a long day of working at a law firm 2.9 miles away on the same street the race is run. I changed at the firm, drove down the street about a mile, and parked at a gas station. I then used the remaining distance to get my muscles prepped. For most distances over a half marathon, I do next to no warm-up. I have miles and miles to get up to cruising speed. But for a mile, for a guy who is not a miler, I need as much warm-up as possible.

This race will forever be seared into my mind as being run on an equally-searing 90-degree day. Hazy and humid as Pennsylvania summers can be, the air was pregnant with water. Front Street had just been paved and was smoother than most all-purpose tracks. It was also blacker than Satan's soul and had absorbed every ounce of sunlight for the past twelve hours. Looking down the street, one could see those radiating waves of hotness that every third-rate director uses to show you how hot the surface of the road is when his protagonist is dying of thirst in the desert. Except here, hundreds of people were going to willing sprint on it, nearly melting their shoes, dying in their own little way, while paying for the privilege.

Even with a full street to run, there were too many runners to send off all at once. So, based on age, waves of runners would be let go with about a minute or so in between the groups. As a 25-year-old, I felt old in comparison to the whippersnappers around me but in my memory I feel like I was a child. I recall desperately wanting to break five minutes and show younger Dane from high school that I still had it in me to do so.[6] I knew ideally it would take a 75-second quarter mile for three quarters and then one 74-second sprint at the end.

Waiting for each group cooked my innards more and more. The temperature seemingly was going up as evening took over. Finally, after what seemed like eons, it was my turn to go and I blasted out of the gate. Eager to get a second or so cushion on my overall time, I gave it all I had. A small sign on the road marked the first quarter mile. I saw I ran that quarter in 75 seconds. Fudge. My lungs and legs were adamant I had run faster. Hunker down, I told myself.[7] The marker could easily be off by a few meters.

The 800-meter mark popped up and my watch revealed another 75. While I was spot-on for what I needed, it wasn't what I hoped for. My legs were beginning to feel the heat of the day and the strain of running way faster than they had in years. My heart was pounding. I could see the three-quarter mile marker ahead and began to lean. I hit in 77 seconds and groaned audibly. I had all but lost the chance to go under five minutes with that slow showing in the past 400 meters. In order to break five minutes, I would need to run a 72.9 for the last quarter and I just didn't think that was possible.

A man appeared next to me and I began to use his hubris at daring to enter my vision as the spark to my fire. Spittle coming out of

---
[6] I had a 4:50 mile time in high school while being primarily an 800m runner.
[7] I absolutely love hunkering.

my mouth, a thousand-yard stare, tight shoulders, fists and teeth clenched, I propelled myself forward. Up ahead I could see the clock. 4:57…4:58…4:59.

I strained and almost stumbled. My legs simply would not go any faster. I just didn't have it. I ran the last quarter in 76 seconds and finished in a 5:03. So close but so far. I staggered over the finish line and dry heaved. Fortunately, I had the good sense not to eat anything since lunch six hours previously and nothing came up.

Then again, maybe if I had puked up lunch prior to running I could have knocked three seconds off my time. I missed my goal for the day but it remains the fastest unassisted mile I have run as an adult.[8]

---

[8] I have run under five minutes on two occasions on a downhill mile held in D.C. that was so ridiculously steep it can't possibly count for anything but in my ego.

Race: Tidal Basin 3K

Typical Date: Third Wednesday of every month

Distance: 3K

Location: Washington, D.C.

Why You Should Run It:

This event takes place on an island in the Potomac named Hains Point.[9] It is run in the middle of the work day in the middle of the work week. It is free. But it is also timed and records are kept. One would be hard-pressed to imagine any other race which embraces the free-wheeling spirit of the 1970s running boom more than this. While there are actually three events that go on at roughly the same time (a 1500m race at noon and a 5000m coinciding with this 3000m fifteen minutes later) it is the rarely-run-outside-of-college-track 3000m to which I think most people should treat themselves.

The course is a simple 1500 meter shot along the northernmost side of Hains Point before you turn around and come back the exact way you went. Pancake-flat with the Cherry Blossoms above you, it is essentially an all-out sprint. When you are done, you go back to work, shower, or, if you are one of those supernatural freaks who doesn't sweat when you even hear the word "run," just head about your day.[10] That's one heckuva way to spend a lunch break in D.C.

My Experience:

I lived in the greater D.C. area for four years but only attended this race on two occasions, both which came after I left my office job and began to work for myself. The first time was just days before I ran the Fred Brown Relay around Lake Winnipesauke in

---

[9] Coincidentally, three races in this book traverse parts of this island.
[10] I'm not one of those people. I am sweating as I write this.

New Hampshire.[11] The second time was just nine days after I had set a new PR in the marathon. In neither case was I expecting anything noteworthy.

Granted, the first time I ran the race was an instant PR as I had never run the distance before. The second time I was hoping to break ten minutes but only was able to get a 10:09. When I ran it, the course consisted of more of a loop, running near the relatively unknown George Mason Memorial, along the backside of the Jefferson Memorial, then around the Tidal Basin itself. Those sites are wonderful to see as a tourist but as a racer, they usually mean nothing given you reside in a pain cave of sprinting. Plus, you had to duck under branches of the trees surrounding the basin. As a 6'1" human I can say I almost knocked myself unconscious from one limb the first time I ran this. Suffice it to say, I feel the new course is better.

Running is a funny sport. I went 1-1 versus a local fella in the two attempts at this race. We had a friendly rivalry for other races as well and if memory serves it currently stands tied at 3-3 apiece. I haven't seen him in a decade and he doesn't appear to be on any social media for me to verify that information. At the time, I could almost always count on him being at races I ran locally and, as the record shows, we were evenly matched. I can't really tell you what he did for a job. I think he might have been married and had some children. Or maybe a dog. Yet, all that wasn't of consequence when we raced. He was a guy I wanted to beat, and I was a guy he wanted to be in front of when he crossed the finish line. Then when we were done, there was some slight ribbing about who had bested whom with both of us knowing, given our like ability, that it could have just as easily been the other way around.

There are a great many races in the greater D.C. area that have this flavor. I met a man while I lived there who ran like 222 races in a year. What was most impressive about this was the fact he really raced them. He beat me in both of these 3Ks, for example. He beat me in every race we ran against each other, I think. He wasn't a young chap either. But time and time again these no-

---
[11] This would be in the book itself but its last running was in 2013.

frills, low-to-no cost races brought people like Ted who were really grabbing racing and refusing to let it be taken over by large racing conglomerates and the newer prevailing feeling of everyone gets a medal.[12]

Look, I am not going to wax philosophic about the bygone days of running and its pureness. That is nonsense. No sport is pure. People are what make a sport good or bad. That said, for whatever reason, people in the greater D.C. area seem to embody a lot of that good when it comes to running races. Maybe it is because they are surrounded by so much yuck just up the shiny marble stairs to our seats of government. Maybe it is pure dumb luck. Nevertheless, races like this still exist and you should count yourself lucky that they do.

So go sign up for a 3K during your lunch break and grab a new personal best.

---

[12] GET OFF MY LAWN!

Race: Beat the New Year 5K

Typical Date: New Year's Eve

Distance: 5K

Location: Salt Lake City, UT

Why You Should Run It:

This race in Salt Lake City has been run for 40 years as of the stroke of midnight 2018. It has an extremely simple premise: at 11:30 p.m. on New Year's Eve you will run as fast as you can over two loops of Sugarhouse Park in hopes of finishing before the New Year starts. Even if you don't make it, when you finish you can say that you feel like you have been running since last year.[13]

Sugarhouse Park is a beautiful patch of greenery on the border of Salt Lake City and South Salt Lake. The greater Salt Lake area is arbitrarily divided into different cities which change when you simply cross a street. The differences between Draper and West Valley City and Sandy and Murray and Mill Creek and Holladay and (ad infinitum) is basically nil. Nonetheless, the border of Salt Lake City literally dips further south to make sure this marvelous park is in its borders. If Salt Lake City wants to fight for it, you know it is good.

The course is not a straightforward circular loop as it does have one little out-and-back section in the middle. Moreover, a series of rises and drops makes it a surprisingly challenging 5K. Coupled with potential ice and snow[14] a fast time should not be expected. But, if you'd like to have a little fun, try to win the Coldest Runner Award.

My Experience:

This race will forever be tied to a training run I did earlier in the

---

[13] HAHAHAHAHAHAHAHAHAHAHAHAHAHAHA!
[14] It is December 31st in Utah.

day the year I ran it. In preparation for my solo running of the 202-mile American Odyssey Relay, I created a trot around quite possibly my favorite place in the world: Liberty Park in Salt Lake City. Not just any run, mind you, but a six-hour run, with two small 30-minute breaks after two hours each. The goal was to simulate conditions of running long with short breaks in between while tired and it went smashingly. All told, after six hours of running, I ended up putting 42.75 miles under my feet: an 8:13 pace.

During this training run, I had felt exuberant for about 40 miles before the last few loops took a huge toll on me. In fact, I barely made it back to my apartment across the street after finishing before I stripped down and collapsed on a kitchen chair. I knew I needed calories and I knew I needed them immediately. Grabbing some ice cream from the freezer, I began shoveling it in my face. I wanted something I didn't even have to chew as I wasn't sure I had the energy. When my blood sugar reached an acceptable level, I meandered to the shower, cleaned up, and then ate some leftover pasta. Here it was only 5 p.m. and it felt like midnight. I passed out for about an hour on the couch before waking up feeling surprisingly good.

A friend who was also running the 5K brought me over some Taco Bell and I unhinged my jaw and swallowed that whole. Soon it was time to head to the race and I had no idea what to expect. Knowing I would have ZERO speed, I figured attempting to win the Coldest Runner would give me something for which to shoot. So, clad only in Speedo shorts and shoes, off to the race I went.[15]

A shockingly balmy 33 degrees made standing around in my skivvies almost pleasant. I was also not the only one vying for the title of Coldest Runner. In fact, one runner (whose shorts were waaaay longer than mine) won based on the fact that he wore no shoes. Impressive indeed but I would have traded shoe material for material around my waist any day!

The gun fired and away we went. The first mile went by in 6:31,

---

[15] I did at least wisely wear a long parka to keep me warm before the race. Also as to not blind anyone in my banana hammock.

followed by the second in 6:33. I realized a decent third mile would give me a shot at a sub-20 5K time. Nabbing such a time would have been completely unrealistic for me to contemplate a few short hours prior as I lay in repose with mint chocolate chip ice cream dripping off a chin that barely had the energy to chew.

However, one 6:13 minute mile later and the final .1 of the 5K allowed me to slip in under the New Year with a time of 19:30; good enough for 11th place. I could not have asked to spend a happier New Year's Eve than utterly wrecked both physically and mentally. I think I lasted until ten seconds after the drive home before I slipped into a well-deserved coma.

Race: White River Snowshoe

Typical Date: Mid-January Sunday

Distance: 8K

Location: Mt Hood, OR

Why You Should Run It:

Mt. Hood is one of the most iconic mountains in all of the United States. So iconic is it that two of the races in this book actually run on or around it. As such, to lace up your snowshoes and traipse all over her face is a thing any runner should want to do. Plus, as is often the case in many of the races I have chosen here, if you need to get a new personal best to help your ego, chances are you haven't done an 8K snowshoe race yet.

A description of the course is probably unnecessary. Given it will undoubtedly change, a good summary would be to say we ran a loop which had a gradual uphill for a few hundred yards, a big up hill, a downhill, two short uphills and then a long gradual downhill to the beginning of the second loop. That's the quick version. The longer version goes something like this.

My Experience:

My first thought was "Do these places really save a lot of time by removing the "w" from 'Sno-Park'?" My second thought was "Is there even going to be any 'sno'?" Wanting to experience snow in Portland, Oregon is a tough thing to do. It virtually never snows there, at least of any snow worth value. One must seek it out if they want it during the winters. Two winters previous to this race as a Portland resident, I actually had to travel to Canada to find some of the white fluffy stuff. The previous year we had one little snowstorm and Portland shut.the.eff.down. Like Walking Dead shutdown. Rick Grimes was out trying to kill Walkers, which was easy because they were yarnbombing IPA establishments, and

Run This Place

couldn't run fast because of their skinny jeans.[16] So in order to find some snow and race in it, it meant I had to trek to Mt. Hood.

It's a bit of a shame it took me two-and-a-half years of living in Portland to venture to Mt. Hood. I had driven past it multiple times en route to various other great places in Oregon, but I had never actually been on the mountain. When the opportunity to play in the snow and take on my first snowshoe race ever came upon me, I jumped at it.

Then it wouldn't stop raining.

The night before, staying just seven miles from the race site, it was 50-something degrees way past midnight and raining. Not normal Portland rain where you barely get wet but like East Coast hate-rain. I wondered if my first ever snowshoe race would be a mudshoe race.

Arriving about an hour prior to race time, I wanted to allow myself ample time to figure out how to put on, let alone run in, snowshoes. I was pleased as punch to see that at least the beginning of the race appeared to have some snow on it. How much snow was on the rest of the course would be determined.

Here, I give extreme kudos to the race director, Kevin Foreman. A very affable chap, he also has a no cancellation policy on races. As for this race, when I asked if it would still go on, Foreman said "If Mt. Hood erupts, there would be a 50/50 chance it's still on."

Some snow finally did fall on the mountain but lord knows how late at night they were finding a course upon which we could run. But come race time, we had ourselves a 4K loop entirely on snow. I opted for the 8K, two-looper because I figured it would take me three miles to even solve the mystery of running in the snowshoes. I didn't want to just get the hang of it and then be done.

Because I was not aware of how wide the area in which we could run was, and even though I hadn't run a step in the shoes, I wanted to be close to the front. I trusted neither my ability to

---

[16] Thank you. I will be here all week.

navigate nor pass anyone in front of me so I wanted as clear a path as possible.[17] As the first few hundred yards would show, I wasn't too shabby at running in the shoes. Furthermore, the sky had clouded over and snowflakes began to fall. It was turning out to be a perfect snowshoe running adventure. I was psyched!

I did forget we were at 4,500 feet of elevation and running uphill, in snowshoes in snow, would tax the lungs a bit. But I soon got a little bit of a rhythm. I noticed I was in the top ten of runners and felt solid. A couple of runners up ahead were obviously going to fight for the top prize but I figured a top five finish was within my grasp. Just had to survive the first loop and then I would know what I had in store for me.

Up ahead I could see a super steep hill but that was obviously meant for sledding or snowboards. As the 4kers had started 15 minutes ahead of us I figured if we were going to run up that hill any of the stragglers would be visible. Instead, I saw nothing but kids and adults goofing around as they tried hilariously to get up the hill. What silly goons. Why can't they figure out a way to get up that…WAIT. Those are runners! Why are the guys in front of me running up that?! Son of a-.

I had great trepidation with this hill. I have suffered a litany of odd calf/Achilles problems in the previous few years before this race and the last thing I needed was to tear one of them here. Climbing this hill I could feel a strain on both, so I was being gentle and slow. I expected slews[18] of people to pass me on the hill but it appeared my slow shuffle was as fast as everyone else's run and no one did.

At the top of the big hill we still had some slight climbing to do as we snaked through trees and fallen logs. By now we had also caught up to many of the last of the 4Kers so we had to dodge and weave a bit. As I alluded to earlier I wasn't too adept at that. Down Goes Frazier! Fall #1. Back on my feet, I trudged forward.

---

[17] I kept imagining some sort of Agony of Defeat Wide World of Sports moment.
[18] Yes, I pluralized "slew."

We got to a point where I thought my eyes were deceiving me. More than a few people were sliding ass-first down a hill. "Is this where we go?" I asked as two guys behind me plunged down the ravine. I guess so. Deathly afraid of tearing something, I slid down the hill part on my butt and part on my shoes. Up and running again, I passed the guys who passed me and began trying to track down everyone else.

The course took us next to a rivulet of grey water which I am guessing was non-existent three days ago before all this rain came to town. The sounds of its babbling were quite pleasant over the shallow rocky basin. The snow began to fall heavier. Two quick hills made my Achilles protest. I began to wonder if perhaps the 4K might have been smarter. I then somehow stepped on the back of one of my shoes and down I went again. Fall #2.

The uphill ended and we began to trek downward. This I enjoyed. My lungs felt good, my calf muscles didn't hurt, and I began passing more people. At this point, much to my chagrin, one fella wasn't exactly letting me pass. Obviously his prerogative, as one needn't concede a spot in a race, but I would have liked a little bit of leeway. Finally, when I felt I had enough steam, I plowed off to the left and into the untrodden, much deeper snow. I sailed past him and set my sights on the remaining guys in front of me. About 50 yards later, I fell again. This time, I had run right out of my snowshoe.

I quickly tried to get my foot back in but this was not a simple contraption. Plus, I was inexperienced in doing so. Plus, my hands were in gloves. Plus, my foot was covered in snow. Plus, I was on the side of a hill and other runners were coming at me. Plus, when I had the snowshoe half on and tried to kick my foot free of the shoe, I sent it sailing about 15 feet in front of me. This all would have been hilarious if I wasn't trying to race. Finally, I got the shoe back on and started running again. Just a few steps later and I realized I had not tightened it properly. I had to pull over again and secure the shoe. Now I was angry at myself for not being more prepared.

Bombing down the hill I found I was adept at running downhill, just like in real life. I shifted through trees and followed the path in front of me hoping to catch as many people as possible. We came to the turning point where I would make a right to finish the race on the next loop but on this loop I had to make a left to start it all over again. I could see all the racers in front of me stretched like ants on ice cream.

Having gained a great deal of ground on all of them since I fell, I went into racing mode. There were more than a few places on the course where we were all brought to a walk to catch our wind, even if just for a few paces. Do not underestimate this sort of exercise: it is tiring. But I could tell I was less winded than they were so I timed my quick walk breaks accordingly. I would walk until I was right behind them and then run. Making sure to pass opponents with strength and not look back is an excellent racing tactic. It demoralizes your foe[19]. If I had to walk it would be after I had put some distance between us and they could no longer see me. I passed no less than seven or eight runners this way until I was at the base of the big hill again. No shame here — I am walking this bad boy.

At the top, knowing there were just two quick bumps to get over and mostly flat or slightly uphill for a few hundred yards, I began to motor. I passed the guy who I had veered into the snow to pass on the previous lap and strained to see anyone else to chase down. No one. The remainder of the race was me just picking them up and putting them down. I felt like I had been doing this my whole life, especially when we hit the long gradual downhill. I hopped over logs I had stepped over tentatively on the first lap. I didn't slow to take turns on gradual sloping hills. The flip-flap of my snowshoes became an agreeable rhythmic metronome and I was in tune with it all.

As I entered the last forested portion of the run, which had us leaping over logs and zig-zagging trees on a slight uphill I had walked on the first lap, I simply sped up. I saw one final competitor in front of me whom I recognized was in my race. I went up the

---

[19] VANQUISH THEM!

incline and made the right turn. Down the hill I went closing the gap. I was getting closer and closer even as I could hear the footsteps of a runner behind me. I deduced correctly it was a 4K runner who I had just passed and he wanted to race me hard to the finish. I used this challenge to spur me on more. Unfortunately, I was running out of real estate to catch the runner in front of me.

I came barreling into the finish just five seconds behind him and finished 13th overall. One of the runners I was tracking down before I fell finished seventh. I have every reason to believe I would have been in that place if not further up, if not for the ejected snowshoe. This realization bummed me a bit but I soon got over it. The race was a huge success and everyone was having a blast. What easily could have been a sopping mess instead turned into a winter blessing.

Later I found out that while I hadn't had the best day ever, I had qualified for the National Championship race held in Wisconsin later that winter. So I had that going for me.

Race: Blossom Time Run

Typical Date: Sunday before Memorial Day

Distance: 5.25

Location: Chagrin Falls, OH

Why You Should Run It:

Ever run a 5.25-mile race? Chances are slim as there appears to only be two of these races in the United States.[20] As such, if you are getting a little long in the tooth, or hitting a little bit of a rut in your running, nothing helps shock the system like a new personal best. Be forewarned: while you may set a new best time, this race will make you earn it.

After starting immediately with a small climb, followed by a small respite, you will tackle a 170-foot hill over the next mile. By the time you finish the race you will get that all back in downhill, but you will experience no less than three small risers on the way to that finish. Do not let the toughness of the race scare you away. It might also be humid and hot, too. Wait, that probably didn't help convince you. Just trust me, you feel like you deserve the PR you run here. And if you have run it more than once, you can always strive to do better. The course has rarely, if ever, changed. Four decades in the making, the race has provided the same course for every single person who has run it.

As the Blossom Time Run is on Memorial Day weekend, you are all but assured to have a plethora of spectators on the course, grill going and cold drinks in hand. In fact, while it is on Memorial Day, most of the locals are celebrating Blossom Time, the festival with balloon rides, pie-eating contests, and a whole slate of other events. How this differs from normal Memorial Day festivities is beyond me, but they

---

[20] What's the other one? I think the more important question is "How did you know I just asked that?" Answer: Camera in book.

make it almost a point to let you know it is Blossom Time.[21] Suffice it to say this will be well-attended and you will enjoy some cheering from the sidelines. And I can almost assure you there is some kind of funnel cake at the end.

Plus, any race whose course directions are essentially: "start, turn right, turn right, turn right, finish" is a must run.

My Experience

Before I even ran my first marathon, I had dabbled in a few 5Ks. One of my best friends who I had known since we were five had started running for exercise around the same time. He wasn't exactly the most athletically gifted person in the world and mentioned he would be running this race. Just a few hours' drive from where we grew up, the race was an opportunity to visit my parents and go running with a buddy. When he inquired if I wanted to join him, I jumped at the chance.

Some collegiate friends of his wanted to take part in this odd-distance race and I was happy to tag along. On that day, I definitely did not think I would end up running it three times, making it one of just a handful of races I have run more than once. In fact, I am fairly certain it is the only race where I ran faster each time I raced it.[22]

While the three races blend together in my mind in some sort of bouillabaisse of running, I do recall all were run on mildly cloudy, mildly muggy, mildly warm, Memorial Day weekend days. I actually have grainy videocam footage of all three to back this up.[23]

My first running was a few months before I ran my first marathon. This is also around the time when I had started doing some "real" running. I remember being completely winded throughout but at least I whooped the pants off all my friends, which is all that really matters.

---

[21] It's Blossom Time.
[22] 34:56, 33:07, 32:59.
[23] I think it is on the same tape of me singing Boyz II Men songs to a then-girlfriend so this will never see the light of day.

My second running was a massive improvement and I was only bummed I didn't sneak under 33 minutes. I really crushed the big hill on this day and remember moving quickly through people who seemed to not prepare for it very well. As I am not the best uphill runner, this surprised me. Granted, I did just finish law school so perhaps a huge weight had been lifted from my shoulders. I do recall feeling light as a feather that day. I also definitely beat all my friends.

When the third time I ran the race rolled around, I had moved from one locale in Pennsylvania to another which put me a great deal closer to this venue in Ohio. I took the race far more seriously and was hoping for the same amount of time drop from the first to the second. However, I struggled mightily throughout and vividly recall the major hill getting its revenge from the previous year. It was only with a herculean effort at the end that I continued my streak of improvement and I virtually threw myself over the finish to get under 33 minutes. I then proceeded to convulse in a dry heave having given everything I had.

Then I turned around and mocked my friends for running so slow.[24] Because that's what friends do.

---

[24] Well, I didn't turn around just then. I had to wait a while. *zing*

Adding Distance: 10K to 10 Mile

Race: Cooper River Bridge Run

Typical Date: First Saturday in April

Distance: 10K

Location: Charleston, SC

Why You Should Run It:

One thing you should know about what colors my opinions of races: I absolutely love bridges. If you want to get my attention, give me an awesome bridge which goes over an expanse of, well, anything and I get all a titter. Add to the bridge by making it an architectural wonder, while also ensuring it is pleasing to the eye, and I am going to rave about it annoyingly so. The irony of getting excited about running over bridges is that, for the most part, while bridges make for wonderful pictures from afar, while you are running on them, they are often nothing special. More than likely you cannot appreciate how fantastic they are when you are so close.[25] Yet I still love bridges.

The CRBR traverses the Arthur Ravenel Jr. Bridge, the third longest cable-stayed bridge in the Western Hemisphere.[26] With a main span of 1,546 feet, it isn't even in the top 50 main spans in the world.[27] But, length isn't all that makes something impressive.[28] For example, the Millau Viaduct only has a span of 1,215 feet but has a deck nearly 1,000 feet off the ground. Running across *that* would be marvelous. Likewise, starting at the second mile of this race and continuing for the next 10,000-plus feet, runners are treated to spectacular views of the Cooper River below you and the Atlantic Ocean to your left. Traversing the main deck of this

---

[25] Sort of what I said to girls I tried to ask on dates who said no.
[26] I am not going to lie: I had no idea what a "cable-stayed bridge" was until I saw that tidbit, went "Oooh! Ahh!" and then realized it was likely extremely unimpressive.
[27] That's called "research."
[28] Yeah, you know you are thinking it.

Run This Place

bridge puts you higher than nearly every building in Charleston and you soar over the water below and surrounding marsh lands. As such, running across this bridge makes you feel like you are on top of the world.

Joining you along this bridge crossing are 39,999 of your closest friends. While this means you won't ever be alone it also means you won't ever really have elbow room, either. Take the number of runners into account when you are planning your getting-to-and-leaving-from strategy on race morning.[29]

The downtown party atmosphere of the race at the finish near Marion Square is enough to make anyone thoroughly enjoy a hard-run 6.2 miles. More than likely the weather will be a touch warm for the race but more than ideal for crashing out on the lawn afterward. There are plenty of bands along the course which I mention because it is nice. Not thrilling but nice.[30] The bands-on-the-route ideology used to be the main draw for a series of races but now seems to be a mainstay for tons of events. Nevertheless, it is appreciated.

Given the soaring nature of the bridge, even the elites may find it hard to run a particularly fast time here. And while all races should be approached with how fast you can actually race them, you can be forgiven if your time on your watch is not the good time you hope to have.

My Experience:

I had previously signed up for one of the other iconic races discussed in this book (the Around the Bay Road Race) prior to getting an invite to the CRBR. Since they are on the same weekend I figured I couldn't do both. This happens a great deal in a world which only has 52 weekends and hundreds of cool races. However,

---

[29] Seriously, plan ahead. Then plan again. Then talk to veterans of the race for how they get to the start. Don't blame the race because you thought this would be lickety-split easy.

[30] Kudos if you got the Dom DeLuise-Julius Caesar reference from Mel Brook's History of the World Part One here. If you didn't, go watch that movie immediately. I will wait.

upon realizing the Coop[31] was on Saturday and Around the Bay was on Sunday I figured I might as well try to fit them both in. This meant I would not be able to take advantage of all the post-race fun at this race, unfortunately. Instead, I would have to finish the race, leave immediately, shower, get on a plane to fly to NYC, then hop on another to Buffalo, before driving an hour to Hamilton, Ontario. More on that later in this book.

Because the Around the Bay was the longer of the two races, I knew I would be taking it easier than I normally would on this 10K. That decision was almost made for me when after just two miles all the energy in my legs simply left me. Not known to be a 10K runner anyway, I crested the bridge at the halfway point of the race and decided to save it for the next day. What greeted me as I made this decision was a blissfully sunny day with cool temperatures and the lovely city of Charleston below.

I cruised through the downside of the bridge and through the raucous crowds of downtown Charleston as we snaked our way through a few well-packed streets. I truly was disappointed I couldn't stay to take in the revelry after a race, which is a rarity for me. Normally I like to skedaddle as quickly as possible. As a sweaty teetotaler, the drinks don't impress me and, for the sake of all around me, I prefer to shower as quickly as possible. As I left, however, the good time vibes floated through the air. You will thoroughly enjoy your day here.

---

[31] Which it is affectionately known only by me I am guessing.

Race: Crescent City Classic

Typical Date: Saturday before Easter

Distance: 10K

Location: New Orleans, LA

Why You Should Run It:

The Crescent City Classic started in 1979 during the first running boom in the U.S. Races were popping up in every towns all over the country. Many of those races needed a few hardscrabble runners to show up to make sure there was someone there to record the times of the other fifteen finishers, but there were races all over. Numbers were never a problem with the Crescent City Classic from the beginning, though. The first race had 902 runners crossing the finish line which, during those salad days of running, would almost count as a riot.

Since that time the race has only continued to grow, embracing the culture, history, and fervor of New Orleans itself. The race not only bears the honor of being the first 10K to be televised nationally but, with over 20,000 runners, is bursting at the seams with people running through the Big Easy. From international elite athletes to those there simply to take part in the Mardi Gras atmosphere[32], it is a race which is world-renowned for being flat, fast, and fun.

While the last mile-and-a-half meanders through City Park and can slow runners a touch, the two-mile straight shot down Esplanade Ave, underneath a canopy of trees festooned with all the baubles one would expect in New Orleans, more than makes up for those turns at the end. Prior to that, running on Decatur Street with the St. Louis Cathedral on your left and the beignets of world-famous Café Du Monde on your right will fit the needs of the historian and

---

[32] You will indeed see people who walk the entire route carrying cocktails or wearing bunny suits or far, far less.

the foodie all at once.

No American has won the race since the late 1990s but that hasn't stopped the U.S. elite from showing up nonetheless. In the true spirit of New Orleans, once the race is over, City Park becomes a raucous festival. Bands, beverages, and bragging rights are bandied around in the lush expanses of the 1,300-acre park, which is also the site of the last legal duel held in the States.[33] If you want to get lost in the ancient trees of yesteryear, City Park holds the world's largest collection of mature live oak trees, some older than 600 years in age.

My Experience:

I did not have, what one would call, a good race in New Orleans. Travel snafus had me getting in many hours after I was supposed to originally arrive. A red-eye flight from hell wrecked me and I never quite recovered. It was a shame as even though race day was humid (it *is* New Orleans) it was relatively chilly.

On race morning, I lined up further back than my bib allowed me based on corrals because I didn't think I would be all that far from the start. Boy, was I wrong. People kept pouring in from the sides before the race began and even after the gun was fired. This didn't matter much for me in the end as within half a mile after I knew this was going to be a slow day. I had hoped for a solid 38-minute finish on this super-flat course but when the first mile felt like a 5:55 and registered a 6:27 on my watch, I knew nothing good was coming out of my legs on this day.

I now had a dilemma. Do I struggle through and try to run a still-slow time? Do I fully engage in the revelry that is the Crescent City Classic with its costume-wearers and beer drinkers? Or do I do something in between? As I continued this debate, a couple of things happened.

First, I came upon a woman with a completely hairless head. Obviously someone who had recently undergone chemotherapy

---

[33] "Legal."

or was still going through it, she was cooking along. Her spirit and verve absolutely made me feel horrible for considering the option of giving anything other than my best. I knew I could not jerk around and play fun on this race course. Even if my time ended up being horrific, I had to give what I had.

Second, as I really began to contemplate jogging it in, I heard the pitter patter of little feet. I looked beside me and saw a shirtless young fella, who looked like he weighed about 50 pounds if he was lucky. I had seen him near the start of the race and actually fell behind him right at the gun. At the time I figured he was just running near the front to hear the roar of the crowds. But here he was miles later by my side. For the next mile or so, I watched him carefully try to pick his way through people. Most were polite or cheered him on but only after he had passed them. Before that, unfortunately they were unintentionally impeding his forward progress.

Finally, right around the fourth mile, I slid up next to him and asked him if he wanted a little help getting through the crowds. I don't think he knew exactly what I meant but I basically told him to tuck in behind me. As I made moves and passed people here and there, this tiny charger stayed right on my heels.

For my ego's sake I would like to say I slowed down to run as a fullback for wee Stone Smith[34] but he was simply running as fast as I was on this day. For the next two miles, Stone and I began to cut a swath through runners. I kept imagining I would either have to slow down for him or maybe I was running him ragged. But with every step I took, he was right there. It is fun to be both physically exhausted and mentally blown away by the skills of someone else. As we neared the finish, I told Stone the race was all his. We separated as the lane got a little wider and the runners got a little thinner.[35] Stone left me behind.

The only thing pleasing about my 41:14 10K time was it was a

---
[34] Seriously, what an awesome name.
[35] Well, the space between them. This is no comment on the girthiness of said runners.

palindrome. Without a doubt I am happy with every opportunity I have to run. Nevertheless, I reserve the right to still be disappointed when days on the race course do not go my way. Being glad and wanting more are not mutually exclusive. Chances are I didn't help young Stone one bit. Yet, while I am sure he gets plenty of support from home, I do hope a random stranger lending a hand sits with him for a long time. His awesome effort, breeze of motion, and seeming love for the sport stuck with me.

Race: Peachtree Road Race

Typical Date: Fourth of July

Distance: 10K

Location: Atlanta, GA

Why You Should Run It:

No one runs the Peachtree necessarily to run a fast time. Nor does it possess a particularly scenic course. The crowds are fine enough but the participants probably outnumber them ten to one in most places. So what makes this a must-run race? The Peachtree is one of those cases where it is hard to truly explain why a race got a grasp on a community and never relinquished it. Whether it is through longevity or eccentricity, a race can just often become an entity containing almost a sentient quality. Usually not one factor but a combination of many makes someone just know that they "have" to run these races. Fortunately, after the 40th running of the Peachtree I am now one the tens of thousands who have done so.

In one of the most evenly egalitarian races out there, 28,478 men and 28,693 women crossed the finish line the year I ran Peachtree. Over 57,000 people and only 107 people on one side kept this from being split right down the middle gender-wise. All of this from a race that had a brewery as its sponsor for its first six years and just 110 finishers in that 1970 race.

On July 4, 1969, a bunch of runners made a trek to Ft. Benning in Columbus, Georgia and ran what was an uninspiring race. Someone asked someone else why they were driving a three-hour-round trip to run a race on the holiday when they could instead be doing it in their own town? Those runners were part of Atlanta Track Club, still in its relative infancy, and the race they decided to start was the Peachtree.

Even though it is the largest 10K in the world (with the Bolder Boulder nipping at its heels) even more people apply to register for the race than run it. Nearly 20, 000 more, in fact. You can imagine that such a huge amount of people are going to create some logistical difficulties. Surprisingly, with a lot of planning, the city of Atlanta does an amazing job with shuttling all these people from one point to another 6.2 miles away.

Know that running this race is a tale of three races. Everyone starts out near Lenox Square Mall on Peachtree Road, then heads south past the original starting line near Paces Ferry Road. The first mile is a gradual incline followed by a steep decline over the next mile and a half. This is where you will want to make some time as the course bottoms out just before the end of mile three. Then it is time for Cardiac Hill.

Rising more than twelve stories in elevation in less than a mile, Cardiac Hill is not only appropriately named but wisely positioned. As you crest this monstrosity, you find yourself in front of Piedmont Hospital. But you didn't conquer the hill to die here. You have two more miles to go which include a few more rolling hills before mercifully giving you a long half-mile downhill finish.

Only then do you get the finisher t-shirt. While some races hand them out at the packet pickup, you only get a finisher t-shirt in this race when you actually finish. In the race's early days, even those who finished weren't guaranteed a shirt because organizers often didn't have enough to give out. This now-remedied scarcity still adds a special touch to the apparel and people wear them with almost ostentatious pride all day long.[36]

Once finished you are in Piedmont Park, which is nearly 200 football fields in size with 50,000 of your newest buddies. It is the fourth of July and it is probably not even 11 a.m. yet. That's how you kick off Independence Day!

---

[36] I did.

My Experience:

In what has to be either a record of one of the top five coolest Fourth of Julys in Atlanta's history, we were met with a partially cloudy 64-degree, relatively humidity-free day. Hard to ask for better weather than that in the Deep South. In fact, when I finished, I was actually a tad chilly, covered in sweat and all.

My time was pedestrian and almost of no consequence. Hitting 42:32 put me squarely in the top 1,000 of the race. Saying I took it easy would be a misstatement of my effort as I took it about as hard as I could without having to work very hard, if that makes any sense. I never jog a race unless I am hurt but sometimes I will admit to being a little bit of a lookie-loo if only because I am trying to experience what the event has to offer.

My time was my slowest 10k ever, including the few I have done at the end of Olympic Distance Triathlons. Even if you weren't trying hard, running your slowest time ever for a race still hits you squarely in the ego. But I wasn't here to run fast, whatever that means for me.[37] I was here to take in the event, see what it was about and grasp why all these people deal with the potentially logistical nightmare of running a point-to-point race on a national holiday.

What I found was continuity. People enjoyed running this race so many times because it is the same. They know that they will run through Atlanta on the fourth of July and then go about their day. They don't care if it is hot (usually), humid (mostly), or hilly (always). They want to know that as many things change in this world, this race will stay the same. Well, maybe it will get a little bigger and they a little slower.

But they can accept that. In fact, they seem to relish in it.

---

[37] Heck, even my PR for this distance would barely crack the top 100 and that was run on a far more forgiving course.

Race: Not Since Moses Run

Typical Date: July/August

Distance: 10K

Location: Five Islands, Nova Scotia

Why You Should Run It:

Ever run on the ocean floor? Here's your chance. The Bay of Fundy, home to the world's largest tide differential, gives you an unbelievably unique opportunity. As you literally race the tide, running over land which will be twenty feet underwater just a few short hours later, you traverse a startling array of sand, mud, rock and other challenging footholds.

In addition, as the tides have to be just right, the race is not run every single year. If the receding waters do not provide for enough clearance to get all runners safely across around the race date, the race simply cannot happen. Also, as we are indeed dealing with Mother Nature, you have to be conscience about all sorts of uncertainties. Just two months after I ran the race, a rock formation called The Eye that served as one of the most iconic portions of the area, collapsed. The sea claimed some of the land it has been bashing against for millions of years. Like the Old Man in the Mountain in New Hampshire, time had taken away something which now remains nothing but a memory. Some races have to worry about whether they can close the roads. Not Since Moses needs to worry about the moon.[38]

My Experience:

When you go to a far-flung place, in a different country, you expect you might have a chance to be the fastest person in the race from where you hail. But not me. I wasn't even the fastest person from my neighborhood.

---

[38] That's a tides reference for my fellow science nerds.

Run This Place

The race started with a quick out-and-back to a set of stairs that would be engulfed with water in just a few short hours. We started our jaunt by running across the timing mat[39] and then hanging a sharp left around the rocky abutment. Runners would then head as straight as possible over the sand to a fishing weir, which I learned is a type of trap to catch fish. There, a woman with a flag was waiting for us. We made a 180-degree turn before heading back toward the start. Our return trip would be closer to the water and therefore more challenging because of the softer sand and mud. The first portion of this run gave a small taste of what was to come footing-wise as the hard-packed but still wet and mushy sand definitely added an element of difficulty.

Personally, I had no idea what to expect time-wise from this race. I also didn't know if the baker's dozen of runners who went out in front of me did either and whether I should try to stay with them. What I could tell was that they were all, at least at this point, better than me at running in this uneven footing. I was simply trying to pick and choose where to go without losing a shoe. Sticking to the advice I gave the previous day to runners at the packet pickup, I was determined to not even try to be the first to run across the ocean floor. I figured allowing a good six or seven people to run in front of me would allow me to find the easiest route through the muck.

The squishy sand was interlaced here and there with a small bit of standing water or small rivulets ebbing out into the bay. Also, as was the case in many places throughout the race, the floor was not flat but rather made up of small rolling waves of sand dunes. These foot-high embankments would provide quite a bit of challenge. Imagine a giant rug being bunched up at one end and you were forced to run over every one of the waves.

A few runners had separated themselves from the pack and I could tell that they were serious about racing. Any potential thought about taking home the winning place went the way of the two or three guys who bolted ahead. A small pack of about four to five was a bit behind them and then I was in a cluster of another

---

[39] I am kidding; we were on the ocean floor.

three or four. Occasionally, the ocean floor would provide us with a small stretch of flat, if not still rutted, rock to run on. When I would hit these small portions, I would immediately either gain on runners or put runners behind me in just ten or twenty yards of running. I used these to the best of my advantage as running in the sand was not my bag, baby.

We passed the starting point and even in the minutes it took to get out here, the tide had receded exponentially. I had made note of one particular rock jutting out of the water which was not fully exposed when we started. Now, not even two miles into the race, it was bare and the ocean floor around it was wide open as well. Even breathing hard I could still marvel at nature around my feet.

Up ahead I could see we ran straight for quite some time and it was interesting to see which route runners would take. Some branched off and others would fall right behind. Others would strike out on a different tact and none would follow. As the path along the beach was extremely wide, runners were given the choice of where to run down the beach. What was amazing was how different the sea floor was in so many places. From sand to flat rocks to small boulder fields to more, it was completely different from one mile to the next. I would have never expected such a disparate footing.

There was one female in front of me wearing the toe-shoes which were all the rage a few years back. On this particular day, they very well may have been useful. I was supplementing an older pair of shoes which were ready for the dustbin with a pair of ICESPIKE. Unfortunately, as solid as the spikes were, they were no match for this terrain.

Around the halfway point I begin running with one runner who would become my shadow for the remainder of the race. Meanwhile, I looked ahead to see where the runners were going and tried to triangulate the best course. As I did so, the chap near me would either run behind me or beside me. Whether he was using me as a water-tester, or I was picking the best way to run, he was with me lockstep. Regardless, it was quite clear he was a superior runner in the mulch; I could best him when it was solid ground. It was going to be an intriguing rest of the day for sure.

We passed a few volunteers handing out full bottles of water to the runners and they told us we were at the halfway mark. I looked at my watch and thought, if true, and I could maintain my pace, I was going to crush expectations for the day. I drank heartily from the bottle and threw it back over my shoulder to the volunteers. I didn't need any more and wanted to have my hands free for balance. On more than a few occasions I had an ankle give way slightly or a toe clip the edge of something. Always able to stabilize myself, I now know for certain why the race organizers did not allow people to run the race barefoot. The ocean floor would have cut flesh to ribbons.

Having put one last runner in my rear-view mirror, there was a long expanse between me and the next small grouping. I saw what appeared to be some flat surfaces ahead and hoped to make up some ground. Unfortunately, while I was catching glimpses of the sheer cliff walls to my right and marveling at the water mark where the water would eventually go later on high above my head, I wasn't gaining on the runners in front of me. This entire section was made of those wave-like undulations which just absolutely exhausted my legs. You would more or less take a step at the top of the wave, take a step down, a step across and then the fourth or fifth step would have you on top of the next wave. Each step had you sinking a few inches into wet sand which would then cling to your treads and turn your feet into bricks. This may only be a 10K but the legs were going to feel like they had run a hard half marathon by the end of the day.

Up ahead I could see tiny figures with many bright colored shirts. At first I thought they were drop bags of the 5K runners. Then I remembered the 5K runners did a simple out-and-back starting from the finish. These were not bags but rather actual human beings. The scale of the ocean floor to the surrounding rocks allowed no perspective. Akin to running on the Salt Flats in Utah, with nothing around to understand what you are looking at, reality becomes distorted.

Meanwhile, my shadow would not be shook. I also noticed he did not necessarily want to take the lead. Realizing he was along for the ride, I decided to save a little bit of energy on these sand dunes and hopefully have something in the tank when we hit more solid footing later. Old Wife, a section where the rock juts out abruptly from the shoreline and forms a silhouette of its name, provided for an interesting section.[40] The tides in the bay do not come in uniformly in one direction. Because of the islands that gave the neighboring town of Five Islands its name, the water flows in to the bay here in an odd manner. Rather than just in one steady flow up the shore, it sneaks in around the islands and will fill in areas closer to shore while leaving dry places further out to sea. If one does not know how this whole tide system works they can easily get cut off from the shore and stranded. For the slowest of the 5K runners, some will have to be rerouted because of this tide and instead of running around Old Wife, go up and over a rocky lower-slung section of the rock. There was no danger of that happening for me here and as I got closer I could see that next to the conga line of 5K runners we were catching was a section of strewn rocks and pebbles. Instead of falling in line behind the others and churning up the mud even more I ran next to them in the rocks. It might make for ankle-braking twist but it was more solid than the sand.

As we picked our way through the 5K runners, my shadow and I took separate routes. Before I knew it, as we crested the Old Wife[41] and made a sharp right-hand turn, he had passed me and put a good ten yards or so between us. With a mile or so to go it looked like he was making his move. But he did not know about the mud.

This last section is by far the hardest. Shoe-sucking mud, well past the ankle and in some cases half way up the shin, threatened to leave some in stocking feet. Forget threatened; it did more than that to a few. While I did not run particularly well in the uneven footing, I figured out a system to get through this mess. Leaning

---

[40] OK, I have an active imagination but even I couldn't even remotely figure out why this was supposed to look like a woman. And everything looks like boobs to me.
[41] That's what she said.

forward slightly, while running mainly on my toes, allowed me to not sink in as much while still maintaining some semblance of speed. Because of this style, the gap between me and my competitor narrowed, and after a half mile of that slop, I was next to him. He seemed surprised to see me and I felt I might have finally broken his spirit. The footing became more stable and we just had one more obstacle to overcome.

As we ran down an embankment, we could see a knee-high river of water twenty-feet wide and growing. I gave all I had down this hill and hit the water knees churning. Popping out on the other side, my shoes and legs were as clean as the second we started. Crawling up the river bank in loose wet sand immediately made them dirty again. It also seemed to be the end of my shadow.

Making one final left-hand turn we saw the arch line of the finish ahead. I had lost track of what place I was in the race as I had spent four miles battling my foe. The crunchiness of the footing allowed me to know where any runners were behind me, alleviating the need to turn around. I could tell I had enough distance between us to hold him off, which I did when I finished in a time of 49:11. This is a seven-minute personal *worst* in the 10K if that gives you any idea how challenging this course can be. On top of that, I finished 11th place overall. I think 11th place is second to fourth place as the crappiest of places (especially when I see now I closed the gap and finished just 16 seconds out of the top ten). But on this day, I was happy to finish at all.

I shook the hand off the shadow behind me, found out his name (Abdel) and thanked him for pushing me forward. He returned the gratitude and appreciated me pulling him along. I could tell I had some sort of abrasion on my foot and upon removal of my shoe saw I had taken off a quarter-sized section of skin and flesh from my heel. The three ounces of soot, sand, and mud in my shoe had frictioned off a little bit of Dane. Some people leave their heart in San Francisco. I left my heel in Nova Scotia.

Looking at the standings later I saw that fourth place overall was not only the sole American to beat me but he also hailed from

Portland, Oregon where I lived. Further detective work showed he lived in my neighborhood. Not only did I get edged out of the top ten, and lose first American overall, I didn't even have zip code bragging rights!

You may have noticed that I picked four 10K races here where I did rather poorly time-wise. In fact, they were my four slowest 10Ks. Ever. Some of that is on me with regards to where I was racing and some of that was because of the challenge of the course. All told, the point I am trying to make is that sometimes the "must-do"-ness of a race has little to do with how fast you will run. You often sacrifice time for experience in running and these races are a perfect example of that.

Race: Dipsea Race

Typical Date: Second Sunday in June

Distance: 7ish miles

Location: Mill Valley, CA

Why You Should Run It:

First held in 1905 when a group of men challenged each other to see who'd be first to Stinson Beach from downtown Mill Valley, California, taking whatever route they chose, the Dipsea Race still maintains its one-way course and continues to favor those who know shortcuts (even if the course has been greatly restricted over the years). The race has a unique handicapping system, in which the oldest and youngest runners start first, with each age/gender wave following a minute after. As the oldest trail race in the United States, it has earned every right to be quirky and unpredictable.[42]

The course itself is a study in contrast. A quarter of a mile road leads to 688 stairs which runners traverse in three separate flights with a smidgen of road between each flight. For reference that is like climbing a fifty-story building. Over uneven slippery steps. From there runners go down the other side of Mount Tamalpais into the Muir Woods. After a brief respite, a monstrous climb of 1,200 feet takes runners to the top of the trail, but not before a trail of uneven footing over single-track footpaths, through an incredibly steep terrain. Did I mention you are also running in a rainforest in California?

Your reward for getting through this is being allowed to nearly break your neck through the narrowest of trails before finally jumping out onto one-third of a mile of downhill road to the finish. I enjoyed, as a road runner, one-third of a mile of this race.

---

[42] The registration process once involved knowing which mailbox in Mill Valley, CA would get the entry to the race the fastest. It hasn't gotten much easier.

It sounds like you need to be part mountain goat to get through the race and that would help. But all ages of runners take on the Dipsea every year and the climbing really is an equalizer for many. Even the most adept runners will not be racing up the hills. As such those who are not as sure of foot have an opportunity to even the playing field. Throw in the age-grading I mentioned above and Dipsea truly offers a one-of-a-kind experience.

The race definitely has a small-town feel even though there were roughly 1,500 registered runners for the 100th running. Now I know runners brought up in the age of monster-races think 1,500 participants sounds quaint, but that is a lot of people. Throw in the fact this is one challenging course, and getting that many people to push themselves that hard is no small feat. Dipsea just has that feel.

My Experience:

Knowing this race basically starts right off with the thing I am horrible at can definitely be a bit of a mental block. Being aware my corral, which is based on your age and gender, would have me starting close to the end of the race and therefore running into anyone slower for basically the entirety of the race was a challenge as well. But these were the challenges I was accepting, and almost looking forward to conquering, as I readied myself for the start.

When it comes to scenery in a race, for the most part it doesn't mean much to me. If you are racing hard, especially on a trail, you aren't paying attention to it. Or if you are, you are doing so at great personal risk to your health and well-being. But if you lay off the throttle just a bit, you can look around and experience a bit more than usual. You can see the sights. You can be part of the course. You can perhaps see something you would not have at breakneck speed. That was my goal for the day I ran Dipsea. Push, but not too hard and see why Dipsea is Dipsea.[43]

As I milled around near the start, there was one section which was

---
[43] Dipsea. I just wanted to write it again.

forbidden for runners to enter. When I inquired why, one of the codgerly old volunteers said, without fear of reprisal: "So runners don't piss and crap in front of the City Hall." Makes perfect sense to me. Apparently this had been a problem in the past and the city had threatened to close the race down. Well, we can't have that. Stay in the Porta-Potties, people!

Wave after wave of runners went off in front of me and I could tell this was going to be an adventure. When it was finally time for my group, "Y," to go, I was champing at the bit. When, not even a minute into the race, we ran through a park and more or less hurdled a swing set and slide in a playground, I knew this was going to be a much different kind of day than I usually encounter.

The stairs were hard, I will admit. Not horrific but indeed a challenge. As we mounted them, there were plenty of people on the sides cheering on the runners. It appeared from my peripherals that a few houses had backyards which abutted the stairs. Their owners, or trespassing fans, rang cowbells and cheered us on from those backyards. I was mostly focused on the shoes and butt in front of me and tried to say thank you here and there though gasps for breath.

After the stairs, we encountered the only place where I noticed one could take one of the aforementioned shortcuts, even though there are supposedly a few. I was the only one who took the less dangerous longcut[44], if you will. I am still not sure if doing so benefitted me as I never saw any of the people I was running with when I made my return to the rest of the course. I do know that running through a rainforest-esque section was a complete surprise.

Skipping across Muir Woods Road and a parking lot we were at 139 feet above sea level. The next two miles would take us up to 1,356 feet and the top of the mountain. If this climb was just 600 feet per mile that would be bad enough. But the trail ahead would be filled with roots, rocks and, for those over 5'4", branches to knock you unconscious.

---

[44] Trademark.

One of my biggest trepidations about this race was the supposedly narrow paths and how hard it would be to pass people when necessary. While this was more or a less a truism on the small amount of downhill we had, counter-intuitively, the uphill sections were rather wide. If you had the energy and the gumption, it wasn't too hard to pass a runner there.

When the race ended on fast downhill pavement, I was in heaven. Wide enough and stable enough for the road runner in me to let loose, I passed more than a few people. I didn't pass enough. The top 450 runners get an automatic entry into the next year's event. Unfortunately, I finished 458th (in a time of 1:08:18 after my two-minute age/gender handicap was subtracted). Far from bad for someone who was trying to spectate as much as race but that sure gnawed at me. A mere 16 seconds separated me from my guaranteed entry. Until I found that out, I was fairly certain I would not be repeating this race anytime soon. Now, the competitive runner in me wants to come back, knock ten minutes off my time and retire having run a sub-60 Dipsea.

All I know is that it was worth every step.

Race: Bix 7

Typical Date: Fourth Saturday in July

Distance: 7 miles

Location: Davenport, IA

Why You Should Run It:

The Bix was founded in 1975 by John Hudetz, a resident of Bettendorf, Iowa, who, after competing in the 1974 Boston Marathon, wanted to bring the excitement of the race home with him. A whopping 84 people felt the same way in its first year. There were only three female entries, led by collegiate student Kim Merritt of Racine, WI. Her winning time of 41:04 was over 24 minutes better than her nearest pursuer.

When the U.S. boycotted the 1980 Moscow Olympics, Bill Rodgers, unable to compete, found himself in Davenport. It is probably folly to credit Bill for making the Bix what it is today. But his presence was definitely a value-add. When he won his first of two races there, the field had already grown to 1,500 runners. By the time Joan Benoit Samuelson joined the race in 1983, smashing the course record with a time of 37:26, the number of runners was over 5,000. By the late 80s, with runners in the five digits, it was one of the top ten road races in America. Without a doubt the people of Davenport know how much Bill and Joan have meant to the race as the city honored these two with a statue which runners pass by after they finish. Now the largest non-marathon event in the Midwest, it is a race of tradition, hills, and Slip 'N Slides.

The Bix is known primarily for Brady Street Hill. Runners barely run a block before they begin charging up a quarter-mile long hill. This sort of incline is tough enough as it is but erupting under your feet right at the beginning of a race makes it that much more onerous. Having a huge crowd of runners with no room for maneuvering around you makes it even worse.

As is often the case with a race with a signature feature for which it is known, it is other portions of the race which can be more taxing. After the Brady Street Hill, those running the seven-mile race see those running the Quick Bix, a two-mile race where runners crest Brady Street, turn around and head back toward the finish, branch off. A block later, the Seveners[45] turn down Kirkwood Boulevard. A runner at my pace (seven-minute miles) will experience their first breath of elbow room right around this turn, just as the boulevard narrows a tad with a tree-lined median. Here is where the neighborhood occupants come out to play. That alone is almost enough reason to run the Bix.

My Experience:

When I ran this race, I had spent the previous seven years living in Utah and Portland, OR. One of the problems with trying to train for summer races in those lovely towns is their lack of humidity.[46] I have always marveled at those who can handle the hot weather but I hope maybe something I do they marvel at as well.[47] Regardless, it was warm. And I do horrible in warm weather. But I digress.

This particular race day it was far from as blistering as it could be. It was in the low 70s at the start with the sun blocked by some haze. The conditions weren't great but I guess they weren't atrocious either. Regardless, the people out with a variety of watering-down-the-runner contraptions were ready and waiting. After putting that first initial hill behind me, I was enjoying running down the tree-lined streets and looking at all the beautiful homes and hundreds of spectators.

A mile or so later, approaching a railroad bridge you will soon run

---

[45] I just made that up.
[46] While it is hard to convince many that Portland is not only not all that rainy but definitely not all that humid either, it is indeed that way. So sometimes, when I venture to the Midwest in the middle of July, I get socked a little bit with the weather change.
[47] I do an awesome Mitch Hedberg impression.

under, long orange tubes hang down from a wire perpendicular to the road. As the bridge is only 8'8" tall, competitors can and do jump up to hit the pieces of plastic warning you "TRUCKS THAT HIT TUBES WILL HIT BRIDGE."[48]

Up another surprising hill I ran before seeing the unbelievably fast leaders head back in the opposite direction. In three miles they were already a mile ahead of me. Goodness. Back down the other side of the hill I trotted before seeing the turnaround ahead. Off to the right, I gawked at the longest Slip 'N Slide I have ever seen. Utilizing it would require me to leave the course, climb an undoubtedly wet and muddy hill, and THEN slide back down. I decided against it.

Earlier I had noticed another Slip 'N Slide in the grass median of the two-lane road we passed around mile two. I knew we would be running this way again and as we approached it I surveyed the situation. The water appeared cold and refreshing. Unlike the well-meaning people out with a spray bottle, I had a feeling a dip here would actually be beneficial. I would barely need to leave the course, wouldn't have to climb a hill, and maybe this could actually be refreshing. The dilemma I had as I approached the slide was how I was going to go about this. Did I want to chance a leg-under baseball slide? I still had more than mile to go and I really didn't know if the ground had been vetted properly by the beer-swilling crowd for rocks and sticks. So, I somehow decided that face-first was best. I guess if I break my face I can still run.

Gathering up a head of steam, I splooshed down the blue plastic setting off a shower of water in either direction. As I slowed to a stop, a young lass snapped my picture with her phone. I stood up, said, "Send that to SeeDaneRun.com!" and continued on. I am sure she had no idea what I said and since I have yet to receive the picture, it appears my words went unheard. Bummer.

Onto Brady Street we turned and even though the start was at the end of this hill, I knew we had another half a mile to go after it

---

[48] You just know there have been a few trucks turned into convertibles before these tubes were added.

ended. I could see I could salvage some pride by running a semi-fast last mile and nail a sub-seven minute per mile average. A guy passed me and said he loved my presentation at the expo the day before.[49] I thanked him as we turned the corner and saw the finish ahead.

Pushing a little harder than needed just to make sure I had done my math right, I hit the finish line in 48:44. I was only 503rd overall out of over 10,000 finishers. At least I snuck in under seven minutes per mile, even if I didn't get into the top 500. Then again, even if I had run the time I am entirely capable of, I would have barely made the top 200 and just edged out this 57-year old pixie from Maine named Joan something or other.[50]

One of the random people I saw in the crowd was a woman by the name of Carolyn. Carolyn attended at the speech I gave on Friday and afterward came up to me almost in tears. The gist of her story was that at age 68 she was on the fence about whether she had it in her to ever run her first marathon. She mentioned that after hearing me speak, she decided it was now or never. We spoke at great length and I gave her my card as I wanted to make sure she stuck to her plan. Mostly I did it because I wanted to be inspired daily by Carolyn as she chased her own dreams.

Here's hoping I see her cross the finish line soon.

---

[49] I think this might have been said to either soften the blow of him passing me or soften my spirit so I wouldn't fight back with a kick.
[50] That's Joan Benoit Samuelson if you didn't catch it.

Race: Falmouth Road Race

Typical Date: Third Sunday in August

Distance: 7.1 miles

Location: Falmouth, MA

Why You Should Run It:

The genesis for this summer road race in Falmouth began in 1972. Tommy Leonard was a bartender from Boston who was working at the Brothers Four, a Cape Cod bar. Leonard was one of those few who were into the sport of running when it was reserved for the weirdos. The 1972 Olympic Marathon in Munich appeared on a TV set in the lounge and Leonard was engrossed. So enthralled was he with the fact that Frank Shorter was looking like he would become the first American since 1908 to win the Olympic Marathon that he shut down the bar so all could watch. "Wouldn't it be fantastic," said Leonard, "if we could get Frank Shorter to run in a race on Cape Cod?"

The first Falmouth was held on a Wednesday afternoon because that was Tommy Leonard's birthday. The seven-mile distance was the distance from the Captain Kidd in Woods Hole (another restaurant/bar) to Tommy's workplace as a bartender at the Brothers Four. These bar-to-bar runs were not uncommon in Boston at the time.[51] Unfortunately, the first race did not have Frank Shorter. It didn't even have 100 runners in it, either. Just 93 participants toed the line that day. But it did have 65-year old running legend Johnny Kelley, the two-time Boston Marathon winner.[52] David Duba, a college student from Central Michigan University on summer vacation, won the race in driving rain and gale force winds. Moreover, the race was used as a fundraiser for high school girls to travel to meets. That alone is a notch in the

---

[51] I will make no generalizations here about alcohol preference and the cultural make-up of the lovely city of Boston.
[52] That is what we call a "good get."

belt for a race which began before women could even run the Boston Marathon.

Less than 100 people and pouring rain is not a recipe for a successful race. But the next year had 445 finishers. Then in 1975, Frank Shorter did indeed come to town. He won the race that year as well as the next saying that his first Falmouth was his first ever road race. Be that as it may history alone is not what gets you into this book. What comes with that history is the sort of thing which helps you sneak past my oh-so-stringent qualifications, though. Because of the love of road running in New England and the fact that Bill Rodgers again helped bring legitimacy to a race (winning it three times) the race finally had clout. With clout comes fans and with fans comes a "feel." As Falmouth is one part sporting spectacle, one part festive family outing, and with a dash of sun, sea, and splash just as summer starts to wind down, you can see why this should be on your calendar.

Or, if for no other reason than the fact that a bartender created a race with the express idea of bringing a world-champion athlete to run it, and he did, you should respect that spirit and head to Falmouth ready to run.

My Experience:

As you have read and will read again, I am just a mess when it comes to running in humidity. Heat, I can handle, but humidity does me in with nary any solace given for the fact that I will cry like a little schoolgirl when it hits hard. I cannot say the year I ran Falmouth was particularly hot and nasty but it most assuredly was not cool and pleasant. What made this race even more punishing was the delay of the start when a runner, unaffiliated with the race, had a medical emergency just a few hundred yards from the start.[53] This delay added about 30 minutes or so of me simply standing on pavement in the baking sun. By the time the race commenced, I was already drained.

---

[53] The runner ended up being ok but I do wonder what they were doing, running on the course, on race day just minutes before it started. That stubborn "I don't care about you" attitude of some tickles me.

In spite of that, my day didn't begin too bad. Even when we had the first of many hills to contend with almost right after the starting line, I didn't realize my impending doom. Fortunately, the trees provided beautiful shade here as we twisted and turned for the first few miles. We then passed under the Shining Sea Bikeway which appears to have been a converted railroad track. A handful of people shouted encouragement from above when I would have loved if they had dumped ice cold water. At the conclusion of the second mile I could tell all of my "A" goals were out the window. Another mile later, I was cooked. Amazing how one can push through 100 milers but half of a seven-miler can do you in.

Over the next few miles, I was forced to walk here and there as the heat of the day sapped me not only of my ability to run fast but to run at all. As I came to a dead stop at one point, I bent over tugging on my shorts. Your bib number has your name on it and people often surprise you by using your name to cheer for you. After a while you get used to it but it still feels like these people know you personally. One guy in particular locked eyes with me and seemed to be urging me forward with his cheers. He was invested in me and how I did. His energy helped pull me up and I began to jog. I made it like 50 yards and was forced to walk again.

As I continued to move forward at a snail's pace, a guy came up to me. He put his hand on the small of my back and said some reassuring words. I thought at first he was another runner lending a hand as he passed, as many are wont to do. But instead, this was the same guy who had just cheered me on and called me by name. I had no idea who he was or why he was here. I imagine he watched me when I started to move again, saw me falter, and busted ass down the road to see if I was OK. That is the kind of support this race has from its spectators.

As the gigantic U.S. flag signified the end of the race at the bottom of the hill, I picked up my pace. Almost immediately a cramp hit, well, virtually every part of my body. I pushed on to the finish and immediately went down in a heap. I was able to regain my composure after a few seconds and avoid the wheelchair the wonderful medical staff had brought out of seemingly nowhere to assist me. As I ambled onto the next group of medical personnel, one asked me if I was sure I was OK. I said: "I'm not going to die and if I do at least it won't hurt anymore." He laughed and said: "If you can joke, you are fine. Way to go." But he said it with the thickest Boston accent you can imagine and that alone made my day.

It was wicked awesome.

Run This Place

Race: Run for the Diamonds

Typical Date: Thanksgiving

Distance: 9 miles

Location: Berwick, PA

Why You Should Run It:

I will not get into too much of the history of the race as there is already an entire book dedicated to just that, but let's just say a race doesn't get run 106 times if they aren't doing something right. I will point out that the race is known for a couple of things; namely, the fact that the top runners are presented with diamond rings or necklaces, and the big honking hill starting at mile two.

Berwick is a town of roughly 10,000 people. I would say at least 3,000 come out to cheer people on during the race. It is no great surprise that anyone running a race likes crowd support. That said, it is more than cheers which warm my heart. Seeing a small town continue to get behind a product that is 100% its own is an awesome feeling. This race used to be called the Berwick Marathon in spite of its distance not being quite 26.2 miles. While I am glad it doesn't have the incorrect distance moniker anymore, I feel the town name should still be included if only because of how much it is a community event. Runner after runner I spoke to was running their 12th, or 27th, or 35th Diamond Run and many of them were local.

But it is not just the locals who frequent the Run for the Diamonds. A large contingency from Canada has made this race a regular pilgrimage for decades and have been the overall winners on many occasions. I was fortunate enough to get to spend a few minutes with a few of those Canadians including the incomparable Ed Whitlock.[54]

---

[54] While this book was being written, Ed passed away from complications of pancreatic cancer. Truly someone who will be missed. I would highly suggest

My Experience:

On the day before the race, I was given a course tour by the race directors. I couldn't have been more pleased I accepted their offer as the course definitely held some surprises. Without a doubt there is a reason why many who have run this race on several occasions get better with each attempt. Knowing this course is paramount to running it well. In fact, the organizers put a few Porta-Potties out at the start/finish a few weeks in advance so anyone training for the race can relieve themselves. That sort of small town charm is pretty amazing.[55]

This first two-mile stretch is the appetizer for the rest of the race. Starting on the double-laned, tree-centered Market Street, runners slope slightly downhill through the main street heading out of downtown. Then you slope uphill before turning right and leaving the friendly confines of Berwick. One mile has passed and you will not run a flat portion again for nearly seven miles.

If you read the history of the race and when it has been won or lost, it is rarely done at any other point than the middle miles. Even if you are not in contention for any sort of prize you can see why these miles here give most people the shivers. First and foremost, there is the hill for which the race is known. Second, there is the false summit of that hill, a small downhill, and then a steep uphill again. Following this you are treated to a screaming downhill to the point of the arrowhead (which the course resembles) before one last long but gradual uphill to the end of the fifth mile.

Many times in the previous years the weather conditions for this race have been rather abysmal. It is Thanksgiving in Central Pennsylvania, after all. The old adage about having Halloween costumes designed to fit over snowmobile suits makes us Pennsylvanians laugh because it is true. So for the temperature to be nearly 60 degrees at race start (a late 10:30 a.m.) was obviously something different. I can only imagine trying to summit these big

---

you read up on this man and his unbelievable accomplishments.
[55] If bathrooms can be charming.

hills in slippery snowy conditions. With perfect footing, I had no excuse other than the 500 feet we climbed for an extremely slow mile. As the sun beat down and the smattering of fans with beer and other libations for runners cheered us on, I was simply trying to conserve energy as best as I could knowing this was not the only hill.

As I left the biggest of the hills, I realized there was no way I was going to break an hour for my race as originally planned. Yet, I knew if I threw a little of my back into it, I might not be much more than a minute over either. Being in that no-man's land of way off your initial goal but between two lesser-desired goals, of which neither will make you happy no matter how hard you run, is an uncomfortable place to be. You must decide how much pain and exhaustion you can handle even when you know the end result will still be rather unpleasing. It is a balancing act and a bargain you have to make with your muscles and lungs. I finally came to the conclusion that I should just continue to run as hard as I could without going too much into oxygen debt. This effort netted me a 1:01:43. Finishing in seventh in my age group, I was a bit bummed I missed a diamond award plaque by two places (and about a minute).

I cannot guarantee you will have the pristine, almost too-warm weather I experienced when you choose to run this race. To be honest, the bad weather is almost part of what makes this race so iconic. But I can guarantee the local feel and flavor will warm your heart regardless of the weather.

You may also win a diamond.

Dane Rauschenberg

Race: River Valley Run

Typical Date: Third Saturday in August

Distance: 15K

Location: Manchester, MD

Why You Should Run It:

Covered Bridges, stream crossings (if you'd like), a couple of big hills, single track trail, and pavement. There are plenty of reasons why the River Valley Run has become one of the premier trail races in the country. Through over 500 acres of land runners are treated to a vast variety of trail running. Runners start by climbing the steep trail to RVR's famous Triple Zipline and then returning to the valley. The trail then enters the woods, winding through the pristine Prettyboy Watershed directly adjacent to River Valley Ranch. The final 5K could be the one of the more challenging 5Ks you've ever encountered.

All of that said, one of the things which make this race unique is the choices available to runners during the race. Like in the Dipsea Race, there is some leeway given to runners who wish to not get their feet as wet as necessary. By taking a longcut[56] you can avoid some of the stream crossings and run a few more feet. Conversely, if the weather is anything like what I experienced, you will wish there were more streams.

My Experience:

As we continue to live through month after month of "This is the hottest April, May, June, July!" ever, I can attest that while it sucks for everyone, it is getting more than a little old for most runners. Furthermore, for those of us who have crappy genes, it is downright dangerous[57]. So when the local forecast called for the

---

[56] Remember, I am trademarking this.
[57] I have Gilbert's Syndrome, a liver disorder marked by an inability to recover quickly from strenuous activity. So, in other words, the one thing for which I am most known is the one thing my DNA says I shouldn't be able to do.

highest temperature ever recorded for that date, I knew I was not going to have a good day.

Much to the race director's credit, they went above and beyond to be as prepared as possible. First, they moved the start of the race up 45 minutes. Then, I received an email, a text, and an automated phone call telling me of the changes. That, my friends, is how you run a race!

I had once entertained some designs on a top-five finish in this race. While trail running is hardly my forte, I thought I had a decent shot. When the weather changed, so did my entire outlook for the race. I decided I would be happy with a top-20 finish.

The first half of a mile was run out of the literal starting gates of a horse fence and down the road through camp. I might not want to run too hard at the start but on what might be the only portion of the race where it suits my strengths, I wasn't going to lollygag. I shot out quickly and was in fifth place. Then we turned, climbed a rocky road, turning again to run in a field up a hill and I said enough of that. Less than four minutes into the race and the first two drops of sweat had already made their way down my head and plopped right onto my sunglasses. Today was going to get messy. After the first mile of climb, we dropped through some trail section with footing that could be described as mildly recalcitrant. Then we scrambled our way through what appeared to be a campsite, replete with teepees and wigwams. I had ceded a few spots overall in the climb but, as I am wont to do, gained them back on the downhills. I will never cease to be amazed how good some runners are at downhills (me) and how poorly they are at uphills (me).

A series of small hills, cut through a cornfield, gave all a feeling of solitude, as twists and turns often kept runners just a few feet ahead of you out of sight. As we approached the third mile, an aid station beckoned. I had already drunk well over half of my 20-ounce Camelbak handheld. Double oy.

I found I had screwed the top of my water bottle too tightly to open and wasted precious seconds fumbling with it using my drenched hands. A volunteer offered to allow me to use the tail end of her shirt for friction and I gladly accepted. Bottle open, I filled it with a cool drink and took off.

Our first stream crossing appeared little after four miles. This also marked the second time in the race runners could choose between an easier but longer course, or a shorter but harder section. Ever since I chose the easier portion of the Dipsea Race, I have decided to always go for harder. I don't think the time saved on the easier sections make up for how much longer they are. Plus, sweet fancy Moses did I need to run through some cool water.

After climbs and screaming downhills we were now in the aforementioned challenging final 5K. As I employed my hill walking strategy, I could hear one or two runners behind me. I stepped to the side on one of the wider sections waiting for them to pass me, but none took the chance. I guess their run wasn't much faster than my walk.

Over the next mile I had a female on my heels named Maria who was not slow with an encouraging word. She would pass me as I walked on the undulating hills and then I would pass her on the downside. Each time she would say "come on!" as she passed me and I would stay silent as I passed her. Mostly because I assumed she had her race dialed in; somewhat because I didn't have much energy to spare for words.

Over the final two-plus miles, Maria and I would leapfrog each other. When we finally hit the road with less than a mile to go I thought I would turn on the jets. Almost immediately my body surged with heat. I felt like I had been tossed into a blast furnace. Maria appeared at my side and said, "Let's sprint!" I did a millisecond assessment and realized that any acceleration on my part would not go over well with my whole plan of "Not Dying Today." I said, "Go ahead, it's all yours!" Maria eased ahead of me by five seconds as I dodged some of the other runners in the other distances coming home in 25th place in a time of 1:26:00 on the nose— a full 10-15 minutes slower than I thought it would take.

The race was run, from top to bottom, like a well-oiled machine. While it is a challenging race even in the best of weather, with regard to preparation and execution, the organizers were dialed in.

I would just pray to whomever you pray to that the weather is cooler.

Race: Gate River Run

Typical Date: Second Saturday of March

Distance: 15K

Location: Jacksonville, FL

Why You Should Run It:

First held in 1978, this race has been the U.S. National Championship 15K since 1994. In 2007, it became the largest 15K race in the country. Inspired by the Peachtree Road Race as a way to showcase a city and bring runners together from all over in one place, it has done just that and more. Bill Rodgers, who I have said should be getting royalties from about 40 races nationwide, won the first-ever event and helped the race gain that initial foothold in the running world.

Since then, the race has attracted the fastest of the fast but also kept open a carnival-like attitude. There is a festival which takes place at the finish line fairgrounds and the weather in Jacksonville at this time of year is typically ideal for that. Maybe not so much for running a fast time, but at least the post-race celebration will help.

The race has a few additional charms which add even more appeal. The last mile is timed separately from the entire race and awards are given out for that last sprint. For some, it will be far and away the fastest mile run in the whole race. Another coveted award is the top 10% finisher hat given out to both genders. Age group awards and fast times are to be bragged about but this hat is a badge of honor to be worn by runners for the next 364 days.

With a community that comes out to support runners along a great deal of the course as it snakes through some neighborhoods, there is a feeling the locals are more than happy to share their city streets with you.

Run This Place

My Experience:

I was hoping to set a new PR at this race as my 15k is a very week PR indeed. But when the forecast showed very warm temperatures for race day, I said forget it. I had long tried to race hard in conditions which make it impossible for me to race hard, before finally ceding to logic. Knowing this, I treated the race more as an experience at a speed that still allowed me to run hard but smart.

Knowing I would not be racing the way I wanted, I decided to get a little more running in on race morning. My hotel was two miles from the start so I figured a good way to get limbered up would be by getting in a slow jog to the start. As I heard about potential bottlenecks on the bridges and parking headaches, eschewing a drive felt like a good decision. About half of a mile into my trot, I crossed the Main St Bridge[58] and a line of cars slowly trudged by. Looked like I made the right choice.

Even jogging slowly, I got to the starting area WAY earlier than I usually do. I used the bathrooms (twice) and sat in my corral in the shade. The Florida humidity was already at 95% and the supposed cloud cover that would make the race at least not akin to suicide was far too rapidly burning off. I was doing all I could to stay as cool as possible. Having brought a throwaway rag with me to at least wipe off the sweat from my two-mile run, I now had a completely soaked and therefore useless piece of cloth. As we lined up for the start, I wiped my brow one last time and tossed the rag to the side.

From the start, it all went downhill; figuratively, not literally. A couple of satisfying miles bled into a not-so-good mile and then I gathered even trying to take it easy was going to be hard. The initial run to the start had provided so much fog and haze over the Gate River that it looked like London. Now having burnt off, the humidity was simply stifling.

The sixth mile was an enjoyable winding mile through some very

---

[58] Or the "Blue One" as I heard some call it, not remembering all the bridge names.

pretty neighborhoods. The crowds were exuberant, sitting in lawn chairs, and handing out mimosas. This area provided amiable respite from the sun, with the occasional tree to provide some cover. The people were cheering and clapping with the usual assortment of funny signs. One struck me as particularly original and I actually laughed out loud. For the life of me, I can't seem to remember what it said.[59]

Heading into the last few miles I was so happy to see the Hart Bridge[60] in the distance. This meant I was somewhat home. Nevertheless, as we turned north to take it on, it curved out of sight. Drat. I plunged on, dripping in sweat, and struggling to keep moving at a decent pace. Finally hitting the bridge, I had no intention of trying to run the last mile in any sort of fast fashion. In fact, I had to pull up and walk for a short section.

With 800 meters to go I saw one man staggering. I had already seen people in trouble on numerous occasions earlier in the race. When I see people like this I want to know their story. Were they acclimated and just had a bad day? Were they from colder climes and weren't ready like me?[61] Luckily, here, the runner had three buddies with him (or maybe kind strangers) who were helping him move along. One was forcing water down his throat while two others guided him. I have said it a thousand times and will say it again: runners rock.

I was finally able to pull myself together and stumble across the finish in a time of 1:08:52. This was somewhere in the top 500 or so, which netted me a hat. To put it in perspective, the last person to break an hour the previous year was 209th overall. This year only 138 people had that honor. It was a tough day.

And then I had to run two miles back to my hotel.

---

[59] Pretend it was hilarious.
[60] The Green One.
[61] I wish I could just download data on every runner I pass on every run just so I could hear their story.

Race: Boilermaker

Typical Date: Second Sunday in July

Distance: 15K

Location: Utica, NY

Why You Should Run It:

It's hot. It's humid. It's hilly. It's located in a place that is not exactly easy to get to. But without a doubt you should run the Boilermaker.

This 15K in the middle of July in Utica, NY has grown exponentially the last few years, echoing the trend of races across the nation. The course is not an easy one. Yet nearly 13,000 runners trek to this 60,000-person town every year to challenge themselves. This large of a crowd makes one wonder why so many show up and the answer is mostly because of those 60,000 people. The rule in Utica appears to be that if you aren't running the race, you better be on the side of the streets cheering on everyone else who is. Not an inch of this course is devoid of spectators, sometimes six deep, screaming and cheering on people they know well and others they have never seen before. In fact, the fun starts early as this first mile is punctuated by a house on the hill with a sign that says ".1 down, 9.2 to go!" While this is always worth a chuckle no matter how many times you see it, the residents need to check a map – they are obviously .2 of a mile from the start.[62]

There is a pride in the race which is rarely seen outside of small towns anymore. This pride is nestled deep in the notion that something large is owned by all. To let down the race by not supporting it is to let down the town and the community. Those you see running the race aren't just nameless faces, even if many of them actually are. But you will see the guy who sits across from you at church. Or the woman who makes the pies at the local bakery. They are your neighbors and friends. And for one second Sunday in July, 13,000 more people become neighbors and friends.

---
[62] Of course, I checked. Have you just met me?

The Boilermaker is a race which can be broken up into three parts. You have the long gradual uphill to the big hill at mile four. Then you have the downhill of that hill and the climb at mile six. Then you have the other side of that hill, with a little bump up again before a screamer of a finish. Tackling the race in that aspect will help you break it down and enjoy the post-race party.

What party is that? Well, when you finish your race just a few feet in from the fourth oldest family-owned brewery in the United States, you can bet there will be a party. Don't fret fellow teetotalers, the F.X. Matt Brewing Company is well known not only for its Sarnac brand of beers but also delicious orange crème soda and root beer as well. Now gather like a bunch of Jimmy Buffet parrotheads in the huge parking lot near the brewery and tie one on!

My Experience:

At the Boilermaker I have been able to strengthen friendships which have grown over time with Bill Rodgers, Kathrine Switzer, and her husband Roger Robinson. As the Boilermaker is organized in conjunction with the National Distance Running Hall of Fame, the chance to spend time with the people who trailblazed our sport is rather unparalleled in any other venue.

For some reason I have always liked the 15K distance. This is an odd declaration as until the year before I ran this I had only run the distance twice in my life. Nonetheless, as one of the turning points in my life was the 2005 PT Cruiser Challenge[63] it is not hard to see why my fondness for this slightly odd distance is not tied to the number of times I have run it.

I have run the Boilermaker twice and both times experienced that hometown feel you just won't experience in many other races. The people and places in rustic Utica reminded me of my own hometown in not-so-far away Titusville, PA. It felt good to be "home."

[63] A race consisting of a 5K, 15K and a marathon run in 24 hours where the lowest combined time wins. I won by seven minutes over the next competitor, almost setting a PR in the marathon. This race set into motion the thought process for the 52 Marathons.

In my first time running the race I faltered at the end and didn't break an hour which was my "B" goal for the day. I obviously also missed my "A" goal which seems quite easy at first blush. All I wanted to do was break the record for the 65-69-year-old division. Piece of cake, right? That is until you learn it is held by the amazing Ed Whitlock of Canada[64]. His time for this race? 55:04. An average of 5:54 per mile for 9.3 miles which Ed ran at age 69. Pick up your jaw.

The announcers at the start had jokingly called my second running the "Brrrlermaker" as the reported started temperature was the lowest in Boilermaker history. That is all well and good until you realize that comparative adjectives need to be compared to something. Here, "lowest temperature ever" means we are comparing it against other mid-July temps in sweltering Utica summers. The low 60s thermometer reading might be "cooler" but no one on the starting line was wishing for a scarf. In fact, no more than a mile in and I was already heavily perspiring. Of course, I have heavily perspired wearing nothing but a Speedo on a New Year's Eve 5K race in 18-degree weather before[65] but still.

The problem was, by the time I got to the biggest, but not necessarily the hardest, hill of this race, I was well off my goal despite giving it everything I had. I fully expected the climb to the top of mile four to be over seven minutes for the mile. I did not feel fast, I was sweating, and I was grumpy. Even as I passed a few runners going up the hill, my mind was searching for a reason why exactly I liked the 15K in the first place. Nine point three miles? Heck, I don't even get warmed up until the first six are in the bag. July? Why would I want to run then? Running is stupid. You have to get out of a perfectly comfortable bed and go make yourself hurt. I am quitting right here. I really don't see the point of this sport. There isn't even a ball.

Then I ran a 6:48. Funny what 12 seconds will do to your psyche.

---

[64] As mentioned previously Ed unfortunately passed while this book was being written. Makes me sad to even write this.
[65] As you have read.

Even with this sudden unexpected pickup, I knew I wasn't getting the Ed Whitlock Standard. Some of my goals were still in play, though. It was clear I could still get under an hour but the question remained how hard I was going to have to work to grab it. This brief respite and adrenaline shot was short-lived as I knew I had to begin climbing again. I figuratively put my head down and began the climb. When you look at the elevation profile, the first four miles catch your attention. Once you begin running the race, you find out the hill at Utica College is the one which grabs at your ankles the most. Often the only thing keeping you from stopping and walking are the boisterous crowds, cheering and yelling. Like Heartbreak Hill in the Boston Marathon, here the crowds lift you.

Even though you know 99.9% of the crowd is not there waiting for you or cheering you on specifically, no one wants to disappoint those who have spent all morning clapping. So you trudge forward the best you can. For me, when I saw that my split for this hill was barely faster than the much steeper hill at mile four, I was disappointed. But I knew I only had two miles to go.

Your gift for fighting through the hill whose top you cannot see because of two right-angle turns and crowds lining the streets, is a long gradual downhill. If you are going to make any move, this is where you make it. The last 1.3 miles of this course becomes a congested sea of runners, bagpipers, fans, and the occasional spectator who somehow looks completely confused about what the heck is going on. To be gliding along, moved forward only by your own power, pushing to cover a distance faster than you have ever before is what we live for as runners.[66]

With the finish line in sight I realized if I pushed a smidgen more I would be able to run a slightly faster time than a friend's personal best as well. I decided that extra effort to slip a little below their time and therefore have good-natured bragging rights was worth the hurt. With people on both sides of the street throatily screaming for everyone sprinting down the hill, I slid in under the banner in a new personal best of 59:39. Good enough for 299th

---

[66] Then we immediately dissect our race and find a million places where we could have pushed harder. Runners!

place overall, my time was an improvement of nearly two minutes from the previous year and a personal best by over thirty seconds.

Was I content? No. I hope to never be content when it comes to racing. I want to always be pushing for more. Pushing on both good days and bad. Trying when there is no real reason to try. Doing what I want, like, and need to do.

But I was happy. Happy is a good thing to be.

Race: Cherry Blossom Ten Mile

Typical Date: First Sunday in April

Distance: 10 miles

Location: Washington, D.C.

Why You Should Run It:

Runners love to feel special and when a city is partially shut down so we can traverse the streets, there are few better feelings. But this isn't any city; this is the Nation's Capital! Among the landmarks along the route are the Jefferson Memorial, the FDR Memorial, the Washington Monument, Arlington National Cemetery, the Lincoln Memorial, the Watergate complex, Rock Creek Park, and the Tidal Basin. I mean, come on!

There are a few other races that do run around D.C.'s streets so that alone is not the only reason to run this race. In fact, the main reason is in the name: the cherry blossoms. Meant to coincide with the bloom of the cherry blossoms given as a gift in 1912 from the mayor of Tokyo, the race allows for miles of running underneath a glorious arrangement of soft pink and white petals. If the wind is blowing and the blossoms are flying you can get showered in a fairy-tale amount of cuteness like Tom Cruise in Legend.[67]

In addition, it is very fast course. While many races these days focus on all the extras to attract all types of runners of all speeds, this one really still enjoys allowing people to race hard on a quality course. Food for the eyes and speed for the legs – that's a great combination.

My Experience:

Mere seconds before the race started, the organizers announced that just minutes before, an accident involving a pedestrian and a motorcycle occurred on the course. Because of this, the race

---

[67] I make this reference in spite of the fact a quick survey of ten friends showed none had any idea what I was talking about.

needed to be re-routed. It appeared the course would fall half of a mile short of the intended distance. My two emotions were as such:

1. Well, there goes my attempt at running my first ten-mile race ever.

2. Holy mackerel! It is absolutely amazing that with mere minutes to go before the start, the organizers were able to make use of what had to be a contingency plan they probably hoped never to use.

Even with two 10Ks and a 30K race run in the previous two weeks prior to this event, I was still feeling rather fresh. Nevertheless, I knew I wouldn't be running anywhere close to my potential. Plus, while running a 9.5-mile race is just as arbitrary as running a ten miler, I could tell the normal gusto I had would be gone. So instead of "racing," I decided to simply enjoy as much of the race as I could, while still putting in a solid effort.

As we ran down the first stretch of road, I pulled to the side a bit. I really don't like to have people around me when I am racing. There is something about wanting my own personal space which is paramount to me. I would probably have been terrible in track meets with more than a few runners. So even in crowded races, I do my best to find the areas that contain the fewest people possible.

Once out of the masses, I noticed another runner also seemed to enjoy getting out of the crowd at the start as well. Then I noticed that other runner was Joan Benoit Samuelson. We chatted oh so briefly and then, after running a 6:10 first mile and realizing I didn't want to run that fast today, I bid her adieu. She ran, at age 57, a fantastic time of 58:56. Dang.

The unaltered portion of the course took us down Independence Ave with the Washington Monument in the background. After that we passed over the Memorial Bridge toward Arlington Memorial Cemetery. Before even getting two miles into the race, watching the leaders already a full minute or more in front of you can be both awe-inspiring and disheartening at the same time. I went with the former so my ego didn't take too big of a hit. Heading back toward the Lincoln Memorial, hordes of people filled the other lanes in the opposite direction. They were now running where I had just been. I hoped someone was silently cursing me for being so far ahead of them now.

Down Rock Creek Parkway and under the Kennedy Center we went. This overhang for the Center has always struck me as an odd addition limiting any truck of any large size. Perhaps that was the purpose. But it seems to be superficial, overwrought, and gets far more attention than it deserves.[68] Pondering this overhang kept my mind off the 180-degree turn we had to make a few hundred yards later. I don't really mind these turns much when I am not too crowded. But in big races, too many people don't seem to understand physics and the "two objects can't occupy the same space at the same time" theory. That said, going through the 5K in a sub-20 made me feel a little better.

Before I knew it, we had run around the Tidal Basin and up the smallest of hills. I remember this bridge from the 3K I had run on two different occasions when I lived in D.C[69]. Then the six-mile marker appeared and I realized my 10K would be faster than both my Crescent City Classic and Cooper River Bridge Run 10Ks by over a minute. It is a fickle mistress, running.

I knew three of the final four miles were on Hains Point. I have a love/hate relationship with Hains Point which started when I first began running the Marine Corps Marathon. It is lonesome and fairly exposed to the elements. In addition this portion was always the point where I would begin to tire in the MCM. But I loved how it had the Awakening statue at its tip. That is, of course, until D.C. moved the statue. When it was happening I tried to be civic-minded and express my distaste for this. I went as far as to look up the info on the creator and see that he actually had final say on where and when the statue could be moved. All he had to say was

---

[68] Hey, just like JFK himself!
[69] Which you read about.

Run This Place

"nay" and it stayed put. Even though I had moved from D.C. when it was to be moved, I felt a connection to the statue. Often it was the only thing getting me through this part of the race. So I wrote to the creator, his agent or publicist and told them how much I loved where it was. No answer. Then it was moved. Bollocks. So now I had no Awakening to look forward to and I was actually dreading this portion of the run. Then came the cherry blossoms.

Wow.

To say this changed not only my perspective on this portion of D.C., but also solidified my thoughts that this is a must-run race, would be an understatement. As you run down a corridor of cascading petals from hundreds of cherry blossom trees, it felt like a dream. Or the movie Legend. With Tom Cruise.[70]

Here I would have loved to have been racing. I would have loved to be pushing hard. You see, in a race of this relatively short distance, you should be relatively uncomfortable to mildly uncomfortable for most of the race and then really uncomfortable at the finish. The problem with running so many longer distance races it is that it is almost impossible to convince myself it is OK to hurt for 30 minutes or so, as I will soon be done. My body puts a governor on pain and says "Nope. We can't do this for three hours." The hardest part for me in a shorter distance race, other than the complete lack of fast twitch muscle fibers, is overcoming that governor. Fortunately, because I was not racing per se, I afforded myself the opportunity to fully embrace this 5K of beautiful running. It truly was soft and serene, with sun flitting in and out through the branches, and a slight breeze moving the fallen petals at our feet. I was almost sad to see it end as we entered the last mile.

Now, not too sad, mind you. I was ready to be done. Looking at my watch, I noticed if I ran slightly faster than what I had been averaging, I could end up with a time of 1:01:xx. But I saw no real point. I had no idea what the real distance was and whatever it was, it was not the time I would want as my first ten-miler. Instead, I waved, high-fived little kids and the hands of the enormous-

---

[70] I'm making the reference happen, darn it.

headed Presidential mascot of, I think, Thomas Jefferson.

Another really cool aspect that I don't recall in any other race I have run was that in the last mile there was a 1200 meters-to-go sign, an 800-meters-to-go and then, finally, 400 meters. I am not sure how much that would help many runners who seem to avoid any sort of track workouts at all but I thought it was a fantastic touch.

A slightly cruel but hardly substantial hill with about a quarter of a mile to go loomed in front of us. I passed more than a few people here and stretched the legs out a bit. Even when you are supposedly taking it easy, there is something about seeing the finish line that makes you pick up your heels and get your ass going. It was too late for a 1:01 but I was glad to finish in 1:02:12. This gave me 439th place overall. But more importantly, of the four Danes in the race, I was tops. My streak of being undefeated against guys named Dane was still alive. [71]

So while the wind was sucked out of my sails a little bit, I was still in awe of the race organization. For a race just shy of 18,000 finishers, THIS is the sort of thing that makes a race a must-do. Forget the bling and the bands. If you know anything about racing, you want people running it who pay attention to the things which matter.

Like Legend. With Tom Cruise.

---

[71] It would end in December of the same year at the Dallas Half marathon.

Ain't Half of Nothing: 13.1 Miles

Race: Lincoln Half Marathon

Typical Date: Fourth Sunday in June

Distance: Half marathon

Location: Lincoln, NE

Why You Should Run It:

Like so many races, this event started in that Wild West decade of running: the 1970s. First run in 1978, the Lincoln Marathon holds the distinction of being one of the few marathons which sells out in less than a day. As marathoning has grown nationwide, more marathon options for runners mean fewer sell out at all, let alone so quickly. While this race would be considered a mid-sized race with regards to its numbers, no one would ever feel it is missing anything as a team of 2,800 volunteers (with not a single paid position) pull off a flawless race.

This marathon is the qualifier for the National Guard marathon team. You can therefore imagine there is an amazing military presence on hand who not only cheer on all runners but provide precision to the event as well. I had the pleasure of speaking at their dinner briefly and their camaraderie was amazing.

In addition, regardless of your connection to Nebraska Cornhusker football, you will receive quite a charge sprinting through the tunnel at Memorial Stadium and race to the finish at the 50-yard-line. The race also has an option which I think is very wise and more races should implement if the course logistics allow it. Namely, runners can choose right before the halfway point which race they wish to run. As I learned during my race, this option can be godsend.

My Experience:

This was supposed to be my 149th marathon. Instead, for a variety of reasons, it ended up being my 76th half marathon. The biggest reason for the change was a stomach bug which had been wreaking havoc on my insides for the previous week. A day or two before the marathon I felt I might be ready to run but it would definitely be a struggle to complete the 26.2-mile distance. But because of the opt-out option I knew could make that choice later on.

When I was booked as the speaker for this race one of the race directors learned we grew up about 20 miles away from each other in northwestern Pennsylvania. Nothing like having a neighborhood friend in a place far from home. That said, even without this connection, I was immediately made to feel at home in Lincoln, which is truly an enjoyable city.

As I walked to the start of the race, the temperature was just a touch chilly. Granted, the cooler temps were due greatly to the ferocious wind whipping around the buildings. There was not a single cloud in the sky and the temperature was threatening to climb well above 70 by the end of the day. I knew that even if I was able to run the whole 26.2, it might be a suffer fest.

I serendipitously ran into a runner, Jeff, who had contacted me about running this as his first marathon more than a few months prior. We chatted for a bit and talked about what a small world it was. He not only went on to get his goal (sub 3:45) but I was fortunate enough to put the medal around his neck when he finished.

We were told in place of the normal starting gun, a cannon would be used. When it fired I don't think I was the only one who had to check my shorts.

BOOM!

As we took off, my main concern, as it had been for months prior, was what sort of trouble my left leg would give me. Stemming from a herniated disk acquired during a bike crash, the subsequent pain in my leg had gotten somewhat better. A high diet of weight lifting and fewer miles had seen to that. What I could tell when we began running was the leg felt solid. I could also tell my stomach was fair and there appeared to be no chance of making a mess unexpectedly. Unfortunately, I could not breathe. Like, at all.

I assumed this catch in my lungs would go away after a few hundred yards or so but it persisted past the first mile. Into the second mile I felt as though each breath was being taken in through mud. If this continued much further, I was going to be in trouble. But continue it did, even though I slowed my pace immensely. By the time I hit the third mile I knew what I had to do. I needed to stop my race day 50% earlier than my original plan. In fact, if there had been a car waiting for me at the 5K mark, I am pretty sure I would have gotten in it and gone home. Take away a leg or make the stomach queasy and a person can soldier on. Take away their ability to breathe and they are done. I learned this as a Golden Gloves boxer in my twenties and the same truth applies to running.

While I was hardly happy with my decision, I could now spend the rest of the time enjoying the race. Well, as soon as I could breathe again. Through crowded neighborhoods where people were out in force, I high (or low) fived kids, thanked spectators, made jokes with onlookers, and did my best to enjoy what was indeed a beautiful day. For spectating, that is.

As I approached the fourth mile I heard a voice say: "How are you, Dane?" I turned and saw it was Sergeant Hagen, a soldier who took me to the National Guard dinner where I had spoken briefly. He was running the half as well before spending duties for the remainder of the day at the finish. I answered honestly and with an expletive which got a smile out of him. He asked me if I wanted to hand out medals to finishers after I finished and suddenly I brightened. My day would have some purpose after all!

As we ran along, I mentioned I was going to hang with him as long as possible. Wearing a National Guard shirt, the Sergeant received plenty of kudos from the crowd. Running next to him in a similarly colored shirt, I felt like an impostor. I had told the assembled military members at the dinner I always thank those in the military for their service. They do the things they do so I can goof around on weekends under the umbrella of safety they provide.[72]

While we ran I began to gain some wind back in my lungs. I thought perhaps I had been too rash in deciding to call it quits earlier. But deep down I knew second guessing was the wrong decision. I only felt this good because as we approached the sixth mile, I was acutely aware how I was almost halfway done.

The course has a sharp downhill here and I experienced what I assumed would be my only sub-seven-minute mile of the day. To wit, I had heard the Lincoln Marathon was flat. This is not the case. It is not the Whidbey Island Marathon[73] or anything, and on a good weather day fast times could be produced. But if you come to the race expecting a track meet, you will be disappointed.

Sergeant Hagen began talking with a few other guard members. As he now had some company, I took this chance to thank him for pulling me along for two miles, but I had to back off. The lungs were tightening again and passing out was not on my agenda for the day.[74]

I immediately felt better by just letting off the throttle. It never ceases to amaze me how a little less effort can mean the difference between collapsing and running smoothly. Run long enough and you will know where your own redline is, but it usually takes a bad experience or two. While this upper limit changes race to race and mile to mile, if you can get in touch with it, you can race successfully and safely. In fact, as we entered a bike bath[75] I lost only a few meters from those with whom I had been running.

---

[72] Dinner there is a roll call of states in which designated members of each Guard says a little something about the state, do a quick joke, or in the case of the state of Washington, a full on "You can't Handle the Truth!" speech that was tailored specifically to running. It was, in the days of this overused word, rather epic.
[73] Which I will get to.
[74] At least not until I finished. Then I can pass out all I want. I have the medal.
[75] Which Sergeant Hagen and other members of the Nebraska National Guard actually had recently widened by laying down more pavement, I learned from listening.

The volunteers at this race were top notch. The liquids provided to the runners were given to us in cups with lids and straws. I can say I do not recall ever having experienced that before. I am not sure it is any better for someone who knows the pinch trick[76] but for those who spill a drink on themselves, it was a treat. I do know that with my diminished breathing it was impossible to use the straw. So I took the lid off, drank as normal, and moved forward.

We turned north and I knew this was now where we would not only begin heading home but also take on the biggest of the remaining hills. And as always, where I lose ground on flat portions of a race, I make it back on these hills. I have yet to fully understand why that is; I just know it is.

When I ran up the last hill faster than I had half of the miles previously, I hoped the final 5K might be quick. Granted anything can happen in one mile, let alone 3.1, but as the tenth mile passed and we slipped by the Lincoln Country Club, I felt decent for the first time all day.

The 11th mile and all the way until we finished inside Lincoln Memorial Stadium was a straight shot up the street. It had taken nearly 90% of the race but I could finally breathe. With the stadium looming like a colossus on our right, we made one final turn toward it. A few seconds of darkness in the tunnel and then we spurted out onto the turf. An enormous video screen showed runners running toward the stadium and we could look behind us to see who might be gaining. I crossed the finish in 1:35:22 which was basically the exact pace I wanted for the marathon. Too bad this was half the distance.

The best portion of my day came after I finished, went to the hotel to shower, packed my bags, and walked back to the finish line. I was elated to hand out medals to finishers before I headed to the airport to go home. If I can suggest an activity to get you out of the doldrums and psyched about life in general, this would be it. If you care to see joy, elation, exhaustion, achievement, demons being exorcised and dreams being made, lock eyes with someone

---

[76] If you don't, you should.

finishing a half marathon or marathon while you put a medal around their neck.

I spent the next few hours doing just that, covered in crusty sweat from runner after runner that shook my hand, hugged me, and patted me on the back. These were not accolades for me. I was as incognito and faceless as possible. I was simply sharing in their wonderful moment. On many occasions I had a line of people waiting to get their medal and I couldn't get them off my arm and onto their neck fast enough. I don't know why my line got so long but maybe the runners could tell I was one of their own. Maybe because I was trying to think up something witty to say to everyone. Maybe because my day had not turned out anywhere close to what I wanted it to be and I was trying to steal a little sunshine from these winners. All I know was that if there was a job that paid you to stand there at the finish and suck in this wonderfulness, it would be an awesome job indeed.

Dane Rauschenberg

Race: Icebreaker Indoor Half Marathon

Typical Date: Last Weekend in January

Distance: Half marathon

Location: Milwaukee, WI

Why You Should Run It:

It is not too often that one can run a marathon in January in Wisconsin in a pair of shorts.[77] But doing so on an indoor track, around an ice skating rink, is a different thing altogether. Three lanes of hard surface surrounding the longest speed skating rink in the country are where the Icebreaker series of races are run. The ice rink itself is kept a pleasant 45 degrees or so; pretty perfect for racing. While this race is not the oldest indoor marathon in the country, it is probably the most well-run. Also, unlike other indoor races, you don't have to change directions every hour or so.[78]

Laps for runners are posted on a display on a large screen TV right where runners pass each lap. At the end of the straightaway of each loop is a huge overhead display of the constantly revolving list of runners. Music plays for the entirety of the race and they take requests! The announcer gives updates for the top few runners, as well as when each runner hits five laps to go. There is always something going on in the ice to your left, be it a hockey game or ice dancers or what have you, to keep you entertained. With the loop being slightly larger than a normal track, you even get the benefit of not having to go a full four laps to make a mile.

My Experience:

Fortunately, for my race experience, they opened up a third lane, which was one more than in previous years. Without a doubt, even three is not enough for ideal racing conditions. That said,

---

[77] Comfortably. I guess you could run naked if you didn't mind frostbite.
[78] And no, you won't get "dizzy". I promise.

during the race, most runners were relatively good with keeping lane one open for passing, lane two for faster runners, and lane three for slower runners. But, like closet space, you can never have too many lanes.

I opted for the half marathon for a variety of reasons. First, I had broken my hand just a month prior and my fitness level was not what I wanted it to be. With a broken paw only shielded by a small splint, 13.1 miles was pushing my luck around so many people in close quarters; 26.2 would be asking too much.

We ran half a lap after starting before getting to the timing mat and then I began hitting my watch to keep my splits as even as possible. A fast goal would be 1:45 per lap. A slow goal would be 1:50. As you can imagine, I was not happy to see 1:48 on my first lap. I was even more unhappy when I ran 1:52 on the second lap. As lap after lap unfolded, I simply could not catch my breath. There were a few chaps in front of me with whom I was keeping pace, so if I was slow on my laps, so were they. Regardless of our similar efforts, it wasn't helping my breathing.

As I began the third mile I ran a slew of 1:52s and thought perhaps it was just me needing to get the feel for the track and how people would react to being passed. My biggest concern for the race was plowing into someone who inadvertently stepped out into the passing lane. My second biggest concern was getting run over from behind because the dudes upfront were flying![79] Fortunately, almost every single person was staying where they needed to be. But I can definitely say the concern for getting run-into adds a second or two per lap.

The string of faster loops did not beget an extended burst of speed. While by the fourth and fifth miles I was finally catching my breath, I was not picking up the pace at all. I resigned myself to running a less than stellar time. Without a doubt, one of the worst things about long distance racing is realizing early on that the day is not yours and still needing to go through the motions for another hour (or two or seven, depending on the distance).

---

[79] Top five guys all ran under 1:20 and the sixth guy missed by one second.

Instead of fretting, I decided to simply watch the other runners around me. Make no mistake, I was still giving all I had; just all I had wasn't very much. Naturally, as I was no longer caring about my speed, I ran off a steady stream of faster-paced loops. But just as quickly as they came, the faster loops turned into slower loops. There seemed to be no rhyme or reason for why I would run faster or slower.

I almost had the disaster I dreaded around the ninth mile. A woman dropped something and decided to stop, turn around, and pick it up, all without even a glance behind her. What could possibly go wrong? Only my Baryshnikov-esque skills kept us from becoming a tangled mess of asses and elbows on the track surface.

What did she drop? A water bottle or energy gel packet? Nope. Something important like her child or her soul? Nope. An old-fashioned coin purse. You know, the plastic kind last made in 1894. Was she expecting to make a purchase in the middle of the race that required 37 cents? After breathing easy for not decapitating a little lady, I actually laughed out loud. Yeah, that's one for the book, I thought.

Throughout the race the lead woman was one lap behind me. Well, she was less than one lap but I never could tell exactly how far. Whenever I would pass under the big board of runners it would tell me she was always "Me Minus One." But I had a feeling that "minus" was probably just a few yards at most. As there was no one else who was that close I kept using her as my whip to keep me going when I wanted to stop.

A kick to my ego was when I inexplicably ran my first two-minute lap. This lap felt no slower than the 1:55 before it or 1:54 after it. It really goes to show you how much weaving in and out of people can slow one down. Realize that five seconds per lap was almost 20 seconds per mile. If one were on an outside course that amount of change would be easy to discern. Indoors, it is different.

A fire under my shoes was lit when I hit the five laps to go and was announced as such. Shortly thereafter, the announcer said the lead woman was on her final five as well. Throw in the fact that, if my math was correct, I was dangerously close to running over 1:30, and that was all the motivation I needed to pick up the pace.

Going into this race my lifetime average for 87 half marathons was 1:30:14. Those 14 seconds bugged the heck out of me. My friend Jay, a fellow lover of numbers, had figured out I needed to run 1:28:28 in my next 13 halfs to get that average down below 90 minutes. I was not going to run that time today but I was going to be damned if I added to it![80]

In the final five laps, what also helped was I knew that no one else would be passing me. Being able to run more-or-less unimpeded in lane one meant that I didn't have to juke and jive. As suspected, this made everything so much easier. I figured, even with the breathing problems and everything else being the same, if I had just run this race solo I would have run a 1:26 without much trouble. In addition, for some reason, despite sweating profusely, I didn't take a single drink of water for the entire race. Part of that comes from the fact I couldn't breathe at first. Part was because I didn't want to have to grab a bottle full-stride among other runners. But, mostly, I wasn't thirsty. It was an odd experience that not until the final three miles that it hit me I hadn't imbibed.

When I hit the final lap, I saw I had to run a 1:50 lap to finish under 90 minutes. Not wanting to leave it to chance, I picked it up and ran my fastest lap of the day. Too bad I couldn't have done that for the previous 48 laps.

I finished in 1:29:57 which was good enough for 14th place overall. I stepped off the track and offered congrats to those who had finished and the lead woman who came in about half a minute after me. Then I bolted quickly for my hotel for a quick shower and changed to come back and do another book signing. I was sad that I couldn't hang around but my singlet was drenched and beginning to freeze me. The singlet, by the way, was my high school track singlet. I am not sure what made me pull it out of the closet a few days before but I thought it would be fun to don it here. Let's

---

[80] Plus, I wanted to pass my buddy David Andrews for a fifth time but just missed doing so. See, now you are in the book, David!

just say this polyester did not breathe very well at all. But I didn't look that much worse in it that day as I did 22 years prior. In fact, with no beaded necklace and white undershirt, I probably looked better. Ah, the 90s.

Run This Place

Race: Santa Barbara International Half Marathon

Typical Date: Veteran's Day

Distance: Half marathon

Location: Santa Barbara, CA

Why You Should Run It:

Even though the racecourse is quite challenging, with three hills to contend with around miles six, eight, and ten, this race more than makes up for it in a plethora of ways. The final two-mile downhill, for example, is what races should aspire to be. After cresting the last hill at Cliff Drive, and doing two quick turns through a neighborhood, runners are gifted with an amazing view of the Pacific Ocean, sparkling and shimmering in the rising sun. Moreover, as the race is always in line with Veteran's Day, they take that connection seriously. The last mile of the race has a U.S. flag planted virtually every ten feet. In addition, members of our military are on hand during that mile to give you a little flag to carry with you (if you so choose) for that last mile.

Sun on your shoulders, an almost inevitable breeze pushing you along and whipping the flag, with the finish line easily in sight below you, this race has a true mastery on finishes. It isn't too bad on the starts and middles, either.

My Experience:

I have run this race on six different occasions. My first experience was with the marathon distance which is now defunct. The other five times have been in the half marathon which I feel really is the crown jewel anyway. The last three times I ran the half I did so carrying a three-by-five-foot U.S. flag as my small way to show thanks for those who put their life on the line for all of us.

I have experienced sunny weather, mostly sunny weather and a little bit cloudy weather while running in Santa Barbara. My feeling is that it is punishable by the California Penal Code for it to even think about raining during this race.[81] The course has changed a little bit each year but the vast majority of the latter half stays the same with the infamous climb on Cliff Drive there to taunt you. And it does taunt you. By all means, be prepared for its cruel rise.

I could say more but, if running in Santa Barbara in mid-November where you can help honor our veterans doesn't grab you, I don't possess the words to properly entice you otherwise. Plan your trip today!

---

[81] Although, with the constant drought affecting California, they may wish to pay the fine.

Race: Tom King Classic

Typical Date: First Saturday in March

Distance: Half Marathon

Location: Nashville, TN

Why You Should Run It:

It is a rare oddity indeed where you get to run in a race named after a person who is still living. In fact, Tom King walks around the day before the race wearing a shirt emblazoned with "I AM TOM KING" which is just so corny and boss all at the same time. While Tom is getting up there in age, it is his standing as one of the founding members of the Nashville Striders running club, not his passing which gets his name attached to the race. His hard work as president of the club afforded its members with plenty of reasons to honor him.

As Nashville is one of the hillier cities out there, finding a flat stretch to run on is virtually impossible. Somehow, the Tom King Classic finds the flattest area possible for you to enjoy a simple out-and-back course. First skirting the Cumberland River on a well-maintained running path, you are then treated to a finish near the stadium for the Nashville Flaming Thumbtacks.[82] Tom King, flat course, and thumbtacks. That's one heck of a way to spend the first Saturday in March.

I don't normally comment on the cost of a race as, being a race director myself on occasion, I know all of the hidden costs which go into putting on a decent event. But, while obviously this will change from year to year, the cost of Tom King has always been rather on the inexpensive side. I don't know what it costs to utilize the stadium not only for the pre-race pasta dinner, but also for the finish line and post-race breakfast, but it can't be cheap. Getting all of that for a lot less than what races with a band here and there

---

[82] I mean, Titans. Seriously, though. Look at their logo.

charges you to run on a highway is a darn good deal.

My Experience:

Two years before I ran this race I met a wonderful gentleman by the name of Peter Pressman. Peter is the current president of the Nashville Striders running club. He mentioned he was interested in potentially bringing me in to speak for the Striders' signature event, the Tom King Classic. A mutual friend, Joe Henderson[83], had graciously given me a good review which piqued Peter's interest. I told him to reach out to me whenever. Given many people approach me for events which never pan out, I filed it away into my mind never expecting to hear back.

That said, I did my research and found out that not only were the Striders a very well-received running club but the Tom King race was known to be extremely fast, reward runners very well before, during, and after the race, and the entire endeavor would be an enjoyable one. I then promptly forgot about it.

You can imagine my surprise when Peter contacted me and we solidified this gig. Given 2014 was supposed to be my year of getting faster at the shorter distances, I saw the Tom King Classic as one of the races where I would test my fitness level. Then a painful calf problem cropped up right after I set a record for the fastest known time running a marathon on a cruise ship in early January.[84] For the vast majority of 2014, I was reduced to a lot of horrible running and my plans were often shelved.

The week prior to the race had me experimenting with my leg as I did not want to miss this race. I had, seven days prior, run a completely pain-free run for the first time in ages, and thought perhaps the problem was gone. But then on four consecutive days the pain got worse. I ran the exact same course at home in an attempt to ascertain from where the pain was coming but simply could not find its source or a way to fix it. I finally decided that I would run,

---

[83] Former editor of Runner's World magazine, prolific and talented writer, good runner and a salt of the earth guy himself.
[84] Seriously.

not race, Tom King, and then probably shut it down for some time.

Two friends who are a bit of running royalty in the small town of Hurley, WI, were also running this race. Ben and his wife Candice had won the Paavo Nurmi Marathon in that town something like eleventy billion times in a row each. Candice is a fast runner[85] but Ben is amazing. Most guys who run the speed Ben does are slight and short. Ben is easily 6'1'' and weighs in around 160 lbs. For the day, Ben would end up running a 1:10 for the half marathon and taking third, narrowly edging Canadian Olympian Lanni Marchant by about 40 seconds.[86] Candice thought we might be able to run together as I was a bit hindered and she was hoping to run a fast time for her. So we paired up at the start.

The first quarter of this race basically had me hobbling along with a peg leg. But then, as usual, the kinks worked their way out and I could ambulate with minor amounts of Captain Ahab-ness. This first portion of the course had us starting outside of the stadium and heading out along some wide city streets. Candice and I had to part a little as we calmly picked our way through the throngs. We then joined back up and started running side-by-side. She had a hip issue bothering her and was trying to do her best to run controlled. When I saw our first few miles right around 7:03 per mile I felt bad. I felt bad for me because I wanted them to be faster. I felt bad for her because I knew she wanted to run closer to 7:15s. I figured something would give eventually for both of us.

The race has to cap its participants at 1,500 for one main reason: the bike trail. For roughly nine miles runners head out and back along a bicycle trail along the Cumberland River. While it is a perfectly fine trail as bike trails go, once runners are coming and going, spacing gets tight. The first portion was no problem, especially if you are in the first few dozen or so and have no one else with which to contend.[87] However, the return trip is more, shall we say, "smooshed."

---
[85] And never lets me forget that she beat me at the Twin Cities Marathon.
[86] Actually, that isn't narrow at all.
[87] Except the occasional non-racing cyclist who chose that specific time to do their workout and would NOT just call it a loss and get out of the way.

Around 5.5 miles, I felt Candice begin to fall back a bit just as I was beginning to feel better. Soon we just drifted apart like Tom Hanks and Wilson with almost no words exchanged. As the turnaround neared, I began counting people in front of me that I felt like I could still pass. I stopped when it got to 30.

I told Candice good luck as we passed in opposite directions and began to set my invisible lasso on the next group of runners.[88] My just-over seven-minute miles began to dip into 6:50 and 6:40 miles. I would grab one group of three or four and soon leave them behind. My leg felt, for all intensive purposes[89], pain-free. The best part of this portion of the course was seeing all the runners I had met at the dinner the night before. Waving when they shouted my name in encouragement, I often had no idea from whom the voice was coming, but smiled nonetheless.[90]

There was a group of three runners, one woman and two men, who were about 20 yards in front of me running virtually the exact same pace. As such, they were chewing up and spitting out runners in front of them as well. When someone is running close to my same pace, I always wonder what their plan was for the race. Did they intend to negative split and took it easy? Were they battling injuries that mysteriously disappeared for most of race? Why is it that we are both so far back in the pack but now running the same pace that the ones we are passing can't seem to hold onto anymore? This, non-runners, is just a small sampling of what I think about when running.[91]

A small, looped portion that we did not run on the way out allowed for a slight deviation from the original out-and-back. This section was a winsome diversion, taking runners over an extremely quaint, if not hazardous, footbridge. Running solo as I was, I could

---

[88] This is a tactic I use to catch people in front of me. Mentally throwing a rope around people, I use it to pull me closer. Like Wonder Woman, this lasso renders them powerless. Unlike Wonder Woman, I look horrific in a bustier and Bracelets of Submission.
[89] Thank you, Mike Tyson.
[90] You have to shout before I pass you so I can find your face!
[91] What the hell do you think about when you aren't?

plot an exact straight line across it, to not deal with a single right angle, as long as I kept my elbow unnaturally high for about 30 yards. Also, by running with no one by my side, I could hit every curve in the inside. Even running the same speed as those in front of me I would, by physics, catch them. And I did.

When I am not in racing form and am way off my PR speed it is never how much longer time-wise to finish a race which gets in my craw. Rather, it is the distance left to travel when I hit my PR that rankles me so. In this instance, when I hit the 11th mile, I knew that if I had been running at my half marathon PR, I would have been done. To think I was two miles behind my own self, set just the previous fall when I was hardly in 13.1 PR shape, was rather disheartening. Alas.

I have almost never allowed someone to outkick me in a race. As a runner appeared off my shoulder, I realized today was going to be one of those few times when I don't put up a fight. I knew two things for certain:

1. Given his acceleration and my leg not working, I could not match him.

2. He had been way behind of me at the start so losing by a second meant absolutely nothing here. His overall chip time was still going to be faster than mine.

As such, I didn't put up a fight and let him slide on by as we made the last two turns on the field of the Thumbtacks stadium grass. All told, I finished 77th overall in a time of 1:31:11. But my entire experience, and one of the main reasons I knew this race was a lock for my book, can be summed up in the next exchange.

Being rather parched near the end of the race, I was in desperate need of some water. Unfortunately, I reached out to grab a cup and, totally my fault, dropped the cup. As I tried to deal with this small setback, I heard brisk footsteps behind me. I figured one of my competitors had read my body language and knew this was the time to take advantage of my dehydrated self. Suddenly, a hand appeared almost over my shoulder holding a water cup.

"Here!" exclaimed the volunteer whose cup I had just missed. I was dumbstruck. This fella had taken the time to grab another glass and then sprint after me because *I* had messed up and missed the hand-off.[92] When you have run hundreds of races, things like this stick in your mind for a long time.

Post-race, lunching with running friends, some of whom I had known for quite some time but had never met, it was great to go over the race with them. One was the race director for a race that I would have included in this book but I haven't yet run it. As I feel it will eventually make the list of must-run races when I finally do, let me give a small plug to the Flying Monkey Marathon in Tennessee.[93]

---

[92] I thanked him profusely which I am sure came out as "Fankewe berry dunch" in my dry mouth, running hard phase.
[93] Look at the bonus races, I, your author, am giving to you. This one's on the house.

Race: Little Grand Canyon Half Marathon

Typical Date: First Saturday in September

Distance: Half Marathon

Location: Price, UT

Why You Should Run It:

If you want to experience the Grand Canyon on a slightly smaller scale, without all the hassle of actually getting to the Grand Canyon, this is the way to go. While there is a marathon, half, and 10K on the race schedule, the best of the three is the half marathon. Almost the entirety of the course is run on a forgiving dirt road on a gentle downward slope. But if it was just a dirt road heading downward, it wouldn't make this book. No, the Little Grand Canyon Half has runners running through a rock valley with sheer cliffs on either side reminiscent of a smaller version of the Grand Canyon; hence its name.

On top of the gorgeous natural rock formations, runners are treated to pictographs on the walls of the canyon as well. While much harder to see during the actual race, these ancient paintings by Native Americans dot the walls of the canyons throughout. It is as if Earth's ancient ancestors are putting on an art exhibition for you during the middle of your race.

A unique touch done by the race organizers is the countdown, instead of up, of race miles. You get that nasty .1 of a mile out of the way at first and then get to watch the miles melt beneath your feet. Not fun to see "12 miles to go", at first, but sure is delightful to see the numbers shrink.

My Experience:

I have had the distinct pleasure of running both the half marathon and the marathon for this race in consecutive years. I decided to do the half on the second year as I was recovering from a nasty bicycle accident and my miles were lower than I would have wanted for 26.2 miles. On both occasions I was fortunate enough to cross the finish line first and set the course record. Both records have since been broken but it was sweet to have my name at the top for a minute or two. Even during those victories, I still found myself taking in the unbelievable scenery. The visuals of a race have to be beyond stellar to pull me out of my blinders during a race; especially one where I am fighting to win.

Even though it is the high desert, the temperature and lack of humidity are almost ideal for running solid times. Sweat just wicks away here and while you are often exposed to the elements, the high cliff walls do provide some shade later in the race. None of the events have a plethora of people running, so when I was racing it was often alone. In fact, both races I won, I was not leading very late in the race. Some of my proudest moments in racing come from having to crawl back and win after having relinquished the lead.

I did beg the race directors to have a finish line tape for me to break, though. Winning a race feels so much better if some string is across your chest when you do. Us mortals only get to do it so often.

Race: Newport Half Marathon

Typical Date: Second Sunday in October

Distance: Half marathon

Location: Newport, RI

Why You Should Run It:

We often read about waves crashing along the shore but I can count on one hand the number of times those sounds actually have seeped into my consciousness as a force above sound itself. During the Newport Marathon, I was astounded during the first half of the race as my senses were overloaded with not only the sound of the waves from the Atlantic assaulting the coastline but also the misty spray wafting over my face. Putting that together with just an absolute gorgeous allotment of homes, each looking as if they were an accredited college, on one side and the vastness of the ocean on the other, I can say this portion of the race was one of the reasons why I wanted to write this book. Throw in sandy retreats named Gooseberry and Baileys Beach and it's too fun not to talk about it.

While the second half of the marathon is nothing to shake a stick at, it is this first half which simply takes the cake. There is a doozy of a hill to start your race off and then a few toughies before the 12th mile roller coaster downhill to the finish, but, even after leaving the beach, the jaunts through tree-lined autumn-tinged streets more than make up for the extra effort.

Furthermore, the citizens of Newport come out of their homes to really cheer on the runners. This is an oft-repeated theme in this book as I truly feel this gives any race a leg up over others in a race-saturated world. Instead of simply sleeping in and letting the nuisance of runners pass by their houses, these residents are actually involved. Any time I am home in any of the cities I have lived in and a race of any size has gone by where I live, I have volunteered, cheered people on, or gone out and paced friends. It just feels like the right thing to do. Here in Newport, there is a genuine feeling that you are welcome and revered and that extra energy helps you when your legs get a tad tired.

My Experience:

The day prior to running this race I had run a marathon in Hartford, Connecticut. I had a great first 18 miles and then, I later learned, partially tore my Achilles. At the time I thought I had simply strained my calf. I forced myself to get a rigorous massage that evening, and doing so made me feel I could attempt the race in Rhode Island. Even if it was way slower than I had planned, it felt possible. If I had known what I had done, I would have never even have thought of running this marathon. But run it I did and took at least some heed in slowing my pace greatly.

As such, it allowed me to fully experience what the race had to offer from a visual standpoint. Rarely if ever have I been so taken aback by something that surrounded me during the race. It is without effort to be a little bit jealous of the people who get to call this area their front yard. Forget the multi-million dollar homes that crowd the area; any runner would be lucky to simply run up and down the stretch alongside the ocean. Without a doubt, while I was quite hobbled, I enjoyed virtually every second running here.

I eventually finished the marathon in one of my slowest times ever.[94] I was hobbled and exhausted. At the time I had gotten news that my father was in really bad health and probably only had months to live. As you can see it was hardly a good race for me in any respect. Yet, in spite of all of that, I remember it fondly as a race that anyone should desire to run. It's easy to enjoy races where you run fast or have good memories tied to them. But when they overcome the opposite of all that, well, that is extraordinarily telling.[95]

---

[94] My 151st out of 161.
[95] I seriously need to be getting some sort of kickback from these races for these glowing appraisals.

The Tweeners: Not 13.1; Not 26.2

Race: Fuego y Aqua

Typical Date: First Saturday in February

Distance: 25K

Location: Isla de Ometepe, Nicaragua

Why You Should Run It:

Normally if a race has sister races on the same weekend, I am picking one of them for a specific reason. For the Fuego y Aqua series of races, it is hard to pick one particular one to highlight. They all encompass the same spirit and the same desire to push your limits so I will briefly touch on them all.

The races were created by Josue Stephens, the son of American missionaries in Nicaragua, who designed the races to give back to the community in a variety of different ways. While all races present unique challenges, it is the adventure race which was actually built to specifically help the locals. On the island of Ometepe, which is actually two volcanoes, many of the tasks the adventure racers must accomplish are what we would call chores. They change from year to year but imagine not only racing but helping those in serious need of assistance.[96]

But come prepared. Even the 25K race, the smallest of the events, will challenge your running, climbing, and surviving skills quite extensively. Do not think this is a dangerous race. Rather it is a challenge where you had better do your homework and train hard to complete. This is not a fun run for the uninitiated.

My Experience:

Whew. That was a toughie.

Originally planned as just the starter event for a very cool run I

---

[96] I'd be remiss to not at least mention some which included: carrying firewood, transporting chickens, and cleaning beaches.

wanted to do in Panama[97], I can say I was not expecting what the race threw at me. Granted, living and training in Portland, I was in no way acclimated to the heat and humidity of Nicaragua, no matter how much I prepared. Yet, in spite of all of that, I had been one of the top few runners when we hit the mountain. Then, like in no other race before, I had the bottom fall out from underneath me.

I will spare you the broken record of me wondering if I would ever actually make it to the top and say I felt lethargic, embarrassed, and just plain useless. I had to pull over to the side of the trail and just lie on my back gasping for breath on no less than three occasions. There was very little room to actually do this so imagine me crashed out in some vines and vegetation, attempting to keep my legs out of the way of those who were trying to climb the hill. Other runners offered aid and assistance but I had no idea what I needed. I had water. I had electrolytes. I was simply wrecked. In fact, I really thought I might end up being dead last. When I was able to get going again it was only because of the promise of cool liquid at the top and then a downhill to the finish.

When I finally crawled my way to the summit, I was far from last but nowhere close to where I hoped to be. I collapsed on the side of the mountain for over ten minutes. Unfortunately, the carrot which had kept me going, running downhill, ended up being almost as hard as running uphill. The decline was so precipitous and the footing so loose, my unstable state almost guaranteed I would end up toppling over and incurring a head wound. To boot, an unbelievably strong wind whipped across the face of the descent with such force I felt like a kite.

After a bit of time, I was able to regain my composure and make my way down the treacherous scree. The heat of the day continued to bake me. An impromptu aid station put on by friends of one of the runners appeared out of nowhere just a few miles from the finish. One of them gave me an entire Gatorade bottle which I downed in one long draught. I proceeded to once again lie down under

---

[97] Which I had to cancel just the day before I was going to run it because of, let's just say, "border issues".

the shade of a withered tree. To this day I have never been so destroyed from a race which, in theory, should not have punished me as hard as it did.

Finally, after much cajoling to my legs, I started to trot again. I knew I needed to get to the finish. Down a dusty rutted road I ran, dodging cattle being led from one field to another by villagers, and doing my best to pick my feet up over the roots, rocks, and natural debris strewn all over. After an undetermined amount of time I finally shot out of the trail and onto the village roads. I only had half a mile until I was done. Originally planning to take around 2-2.5 hours for this course (which was probably closer to 30K), I didn't even crack four hours. Also, instead of finishing dead last as I felt I might, I finished almost statistically in the middle (52nd out of 98). But my favorite interaction happened outside of the race.

Throughout the previous day I had ventured into a small market to buy water and Coke. Each time I gave the woman inside more than what she was charging for the drink (mostly because what she was charging was way too little). Knowing I did not have the energy to make it back to my room after this race, even though it was just a five-minute walk, I stumbled into this market, just a block away from the finish. Thinking my small acts of generosity earlier would by me some credit (I had no money on me) I hobbled to the store and asked for a Coke. I explained I would come back soon with the money, hoping she would believe me. The shopkeeper could not have been happier to extend me the courtesy and in fact tried to tell me I did not have to pay. I waved off this notion and even though it took me more than a few hours to make it back to her shop, I definitely paid her back. Here was someone, with way too little, who found it no problem whatsoever to give something to someone who obviously had way more than her.

Long after the disappointment of this race and later the cancelation of my Panama run fades, I will remember that kindness.

Race: Jupiter Peak Steeplechase

Typical Date: Second Saturday in July

Distance: 16-ish miles

Location: Park City, UT

Why You Should Run It:

Climbing 3,000 feet in eight miles is hard. When you start said climb already 7,000 feet above sea level, it gets much harder. But running in the clean air of Park City, UT, with the peak of a mountain serving as your halfway point, is well worth the effort it takes.

The Jupiter Peak Steeplechase was often run right around the time of the great Outdoor Retailer show held in Salt Lake City a few dozen miles away. The show has since moved to Denver as a protest to the stances the Trump administration, and subsequently Utah government, took towards national lands. For many reasons this is a disappointment but one which affects this race is how normal mortals would often be running against some of the greatest trail runners in the country who just happened by to take on a challenge. Watching these half-billy-goat humans scamper up a cliff face while you suck wind and try not to trip was half the fun. Granted, more than a few of these hybrid runners still live in the area or travel to the race nonetheless, so the awe-inspiring runs of others is not completely gone.

My Experience:

Right off the bat, you start running up. I barely feel human until six miles into any race, so starting off with a steeply vertical climb, after standing still at 7,000 feet, means I will be in for a test. I have always said it is paramount to know one's own weaknesses. The next best thing to do is to work on those weaknesses. For me, one major weakness is uphill running on trails. I am terrible at it. It doesn't behoove me much to spend a great deal of time doing it as I don't really race trails that much. Nevertheless, I have created this Galloway-esque run-walk method which usually keeps me right in the thick of things while others are purely "running." I started using this almost immediately out of the chute, allowing many others to stream by. This method would haunt me a little bit later.

While a tad sunny and warm at the start, I knew the weather would get cooler on the backside of the mountain, as well as the fact we would be three-quarters of a mile higher. After about eight minutes of run/jog/hiking, the course made a right-hand turn off the gravelly road we were on and then started onto the single-track trail which would comprise more than 90% of the course from there on out. For those not in the know, this single-track trail makes it virtually impossible to pass another runner without encountering uneven footing, possibly a stray elbow, and maybe a branch or two to the face.[98]

I soon realized how taking it "easy" at the beginning had saved my lungs and legs for the latter portions of the climb to the top, as well as the descent to come. Unfortunately, it also put me into the conga line of runners with very little room for escape. Occasionally, I could find a spare inch to dart past a few runners, but hoped the rest of the climb would have some wider road portions where that would be easier.

My plan was to get to the Jupiter Peak halfway point in about 90 minutes and then hopefully come back down in 60 minutes for an even two-and-a-half hours. I knew doing so would put me nowhere close to the leaders but would indeed be a good time for me.

About six miles into the run, right on schedule, I felt better to the umpteenth degree; my breathing stabilized and I didn't walk another step until the base of Jupiter Peak. I passed a dozen or so runners and could feel my lungs opening up. Then Jupiter Peak loomed in front of me. I could see runners on hands and knees

---
[98] The latter often occurs in rail racing anyway when you are 6'1".

SLOWLY moving up the side of this hill, set seemingly at a 90-degree angle against the horizon. Upon reaching the hill, I was left with no choice but to follow suit. Bent over at the waist, grabbing rocks and stones, I picked my way up this mountainside.[99]

About halfway up the climb, I heard someone in front of me mention a "false summit." This refers to how you feel you are at the top but then there is more climb to go, often hidden from view. At one point the climb evened out for a second, and I stopped to take in the fantastic view. I figured this was the false summit they mentioned and continued onto the top. Touching the flagpole at Jupiter Peak, as per tradition, I saw got to the top at 1:26:36. I was ahead of schedule!

As I began to formulate my plan of how to overtake as many runners as I could on the downhill, I could see a few hundred yards in the distance runners were climbing a second peak. Well, crap. The false summit I had heard of was actually Jupiter Peak! This last hill was nowhere near as hard as all we had encountered but we had to climb it nonetheless. Ten minutes later I was ready for the real descent.

Unfortunately, my ability to go as fast as I would have like was blocked, in some way, by other runners who I was catching but could not pass because of the single track. This is by no means their fault. It is my responsibility to either let them know I want to pass and they will step to the side, or I simply have to go around. On this course, there wasn't much space to go around and since we were descending at such a great speed, I did not think it was right to ask anyone to step aside.

So I bided my time and just tried to enjoy the absolutely gorgeous scenery all the while picking places to make a move. I began to feel a blister forming on my left heel which I sometimes get running on the flattest of roads. It simply seems to be a by-product of my running style/stride and I can often change something to alleviate the pressure. In this race I had no choice but to ignore it given the screaming downhill nature of the course.

---

[99] There is a portion, albeit small, that is at a 55% incline. That's ridiculous.

I continued to pick runners off and finally could see the town below, not too far away. There were a few mountain cyclists on the trail which we could have done without but most were pleasant and moved their bikes to the side. I can say this entire downhill felt like one wonderfully controlled fall, even if I knew my quads were taking a beating. Enjoying the scenery was only done in small glimpses as well, since in this kind of race, if you look at it too much, you become part of it.

Before what felt like far less distance and time than had actually passed, we suddenly burst forth from the trail and onto a paved road. For about 200 yards, pavement allowed us road runners just about a minute of time to show what we could do. I felt bad passing two more runners in this short stretch but having tip-toed through a great deal of the single-track trail previously, I was mildly vindicated. Every section is part of the entire race, after all. You have to be ready to run everything in front of you.

Just a little bit off of my descent goal with a 1:01:52 second half, I was still able to eke out a 2:28:29, good enough for 47th place overall in the male division. Four superb women beat me to the line, keeping me just out of the top 50 overall. Dastardly ladies.

Race: Goodwater Trail Race

Typical Date: Late January

Distance: 16-ish miles

Location: Georgetown, TX

Why You Should Run It:

A litany of events are held on the days surrounding this race, including a short eight-mile version of the race I am recommending; a marathon; and a double marathon which could be done by a team or solo. Over an extremely challenging course, circumnavigating Lake Georgetown, any distance would be worthy of bragging about its completion. For me, the 16-mile distance was just long enough to really put some miles on my legs without beginning to border on the extreme. Given how laborious the footing was on this all-trail course, I think that was definitely the safest option.

There will likely be no one to cheer you on at this race. The first aid station you encounter is a serve-yourself variety. Four miles after that is the unceremonious turnaround with another aid station. As it is January in Texas, the weather should be fine for you to get along on those aid stations alone but I would highly suggest bringing a handheld or hydration pack. You may wish for your hands to be free for stabilization and to keep yourself upright, so I went with a pack. The forest and trail are taxing, but provide a sense of wildness because of that entire lack of spectators along the course thing. A remote, almost primal sense accompanies you as you take on the elements and occasionally another competitor. This course is definitely one you do if for no other reason than to massage your ego into thinking you are a bad ass.

My Experience:

From the start of the race, which began in the grass median of the parking lot and immediately dove into the woods on a crushed gravel trail, I could see it would be very hard to pass anyone at all. In addition, traversing so many types of terrain, it was clear there would be next to no uniformity in the footing upon which we ran. One was going to have to pay attention to stay upright.

Two chaps jolted out to the front and I just had a feeling they were running the eight-mile version of this race. Four other gentlemen were in front of me as we quickly separated ourselves from the rest of the pack. For the next 2.5 miles I stayed in the back pocket of the last runner, trying to figure out who was running what, who was going to separate, and when might be a good time to pick things up. The footing was definitely on the strenuous side and ever-changing. Roots and grass here, rocks and slickness there. I spent very little time looking ahead of me and most of it looking at the ground.

The first runner in the four had separated himself and the next runner followed a bit behind. However, I was tucked behind the next two and couldn't make a move. Finally, I "onyourleft"ed in a small opening and bounded forward past these two. Soon I was the next runner's heels with the first runner vanished into the twists and turns ahead.

In the next mile, I kept attempting to figure out if this runner was in my race and if so, how I could get around him. We passed a section where the forest opened and we ran across some smooth slate-like surface. To our right was the lake below with a rather precipitous drop. I noticed there was nothing really stopping someone if they fell. It wasn't exactly "dangerous" but it wasn't exactly "safe" either. I can't imagine what someone running in darker conditions for the double marathon would do here.

At one mild fork in the trail, the runner directly in front of me went right. I saw a pink pin flag to our left signifying the correct way and yelled he was going the wrong way. He only lost about ten feet but it was enough for me to get around him. Finally, an open trail.

Not long after that, the first runner overall running the eight-mile race came flying back at me. A minute or so later the second runner did as well. As expected, the two I surmised were running the shorter version of the race were doing just that. That meant I was, at worst, in second place overall in my own race. When I saw no one else coming back to me I figured the last runner was running the 16-miler. I approached the aid station at the fourth mile and saw him darting through the trees in the distance. Good. I will go catch him. Nothing will stop me now.

I then promptly went the wrong way.

Running up the trail I popped out into a parking lot. I immediately knew I was off-course. Damn it. I ran back and got myself back on trail. Or at least thought I did. I picked up the pace trying to ascertain if I was on the right trail but couldn't see the first place runner. I skirted out of the trail into a long opening and saw no one up ahead. Somehow the guy I had passed a bit back had not gotten in front of me either. Because of how far I could see, I assumed I would be able to see the lead runner here if I was on the right track. Bollocks. Now I wasn't sure. But the pink flag told me I was going the right direction, so no choice but to push on.

I ran up a small hill and into the forest again, pressing the pace even more. Half of a mile later, I finally saw the leader up ahead. I let out a huge sigh of relief knowing I was on the right course. He would disappear out of view every once in a while over the next few miles but each time he came back into my sight I saw I was closer. He had obviously put a sizeable lead on me at one point and I don't know if it was because of my wrong turn or he was just running hard. Either way I was closing the gap now.

With about half of a mile to go, I saw three people sitting in a field. I thought this might be the turnaround but when I saw no aid station, I realized they were the only spectators. Well, they weren't spectating but rather walking a dog. But one made eye contact with me and that sorta counts as a relationship, like my high school dating life.[100]

---

[100] *Rimshot*.

We hit a paved section and I recall the race director telling us this was the last bit before the turn home. I dialed up my speed and when the lead runner stopped at the aid station, I passed him. I ran another ten feet around the turnaround pole and decided to grab a cup of Coke at the aid station. I was wearing my Camelbak hydration pack and felt that would be enough to get me back. However, given the humidity and how much I was sweating, grabbing additional fluid where it was offered was not going to be a bad idea. I saw the three cans they had out where all unopened. There didn't seem to be any cups at the ready with Coke already in them. Waiting for someone to pour is fine and dandy when you aren't trying to race a guy who is six inches from you but that wasn't working for me. So I grabbed a can, opened it up, poured a bit down my throat (never letting the can touch my lips), thanked the volunteers, placed it on the table, and took off.

Downhill. On pavement. Now that is how I like to trail run! With the runner (Allen) behind me by a few steps, I knew it was now time for me to be the mouse and him to be the cat. But I felt good in my ability to turn it on in this second half. I knew the route now, I knew what was in store, and I knew it was time to run to victory. Like a champion.

slip *splat* *LOUD EXPLETIVE*

Down I went. After leaving the paved portion and hitting the trail again, I was no longer in my element. Right when I was feeling good, I took my eyes off the trail. A few people had passed me in the opposite direction so while I went down a hill on a curve, I looked ahead to make sure others weren't coming. That small lapse in paying attention to my feet placement had them slipping out from underneath me. Ribs and forearm first, I went sprawling onto a mossy slippery rock.

Sumbitch, that hurt. I checked to make sure that I didn't break anything and still wasn't sure when I started running again. A quick assessment showed I would just be leaving behind flesh, skin, and blood. Not the worst thing in the world, thankfully. The runner behind me (Allen) had caught me and graciously stopped to see if I was OK. I thanked him and waved him on. Since I was OK and sure as hell was going to try to beat him, I wanted him to keep going.

Now, more cautious, I began to try and make up the distance. Surprisingly, I was still within striking distance of Allen, albeit further away than I would like. Within a few hundred yards, after picking my way back, I was his shadow once again. As long as I didn't fall, I would be...

slip *splat* *LOUD EXPLETIVE*

This one hurt more than the first but didn't come with a bone crushing hit. Instead it was just a hand slice and some contusions on the other side of the body. Allen turned around again to check my status and once again I want to point out that this was a very classy move. I am pretty sure anyone who has a soul would do the same thing but not everyone thinks about it during a race. I thanked him again and mentioned I thought I was good enough to continue.

A few hundred yards later we passed a stream crossing and I splashed water on my wounds to make sure nothing looked specifically horrible. Fortunately, it appeared this wouldn't require a doctor's visit. So, I dusted myself off and began doubling my effort to catch Allen. For those of you scoring at home, this is the third time I have been in this position.[101]

This time the gap to close was not as large as before. As we entered the clearing when I had thought I might be on the wrong trail, I passed Allen. I told him it was awfully cool of him to wait and he said "There's no room for ego if someone is hurt." We chatted a little bit here and there as we entered a relatively rocky and slick section. Now it was Allen's turn to be right on my heels.

As we approached the aid station with four miles to go as I felt I might be holding him back. I was cautiously traversing the rocks as I think one more fall would have done me in. But Allen wasn't

---

[101] And it is the third time even if you are alone.

in any hurry to pass me so we stayed this way until the water tubs on the table at mile 12.

Again, even though I had the Camelbak on (and had been drinking from it) I decided to grab a drink here. In fact, using the conical cups next to the jug, I took three drinks. Allen did the same and then took off right behind me. We stayed this way for about two miles as the sun began to penetrate the overcast skies.

My cautiousness continued but I didn't hear Allen as much as before. I realized my watch had stopped on my second fall so I had no idea really how much time I had left until I was finished. Since there were no miles markers and I was unfamiliar with the trail there was no real way to gauge distance until the finish. I was hoping to use my watch to help me through a rough patch or two. Unfortunately, that was not to be. Just focus on the trail, Dane.

I trudged on and came to a rather steep hill that forced me to walk. I stepped to the side a bit to let Allen pass if he needed to. He wasn't there. Hmm. I started hiking up the hill and then rather far behind me heard footsteps. It appeared I had started to put a gap between us. This race was now mine to lose.

I continued to push the envelope with one last spurt of energy. I passed over the first road near the start and completely forgot there was a second. My energy was waning. Every bit of the trail looked like every other bit of the trail. Finally, with 100 yards to go, I could see some movement through the forest that looked like finish line flags. Noise from a speaker filtered through the trees. Colored banners appeared and the clearing opened. Twenty yards later I was finished.

Crossing in 2:19:32, I had won.

Allen finished a little over a minute behind me and I made sure to thank him for being such a stand-up guy. The race atmosphere was very relaxed. There was some food and drink for runners to nosh on and occasionally a runner would come from either direction finishing one of the many races. I wanted to stay longer but after receiving my award I knew I needed to head home to tend to my wounds.

Not a bad way to start a weekend as I continued to get very lucky as a Master's runner. I had won or placed high in a good percentage of the races I had run since I turned 40. Placement, I have always said, is just a matter of having people who are faster than you not showing up.

But life is about showing up. So while I know that on any given day I am not the fastest runner out there, I can only get to the finish by being at the start.

Race: Around the Bay Road Race

Typical Date: First Sunday in April

Distance: 30K

Location: Hamilton ON

Why You Should Run It:

One sentence should do it: it is the oldest race in North America.

Still reading? OK, I will give you your money's worth. The 30K distance is relatively rare, at least in the United States. As I wrote in my second book, I think it is an excellent distance to help runners prepare for the marathon. Many people jump straight from the half marathon, if they even do a half at all. But 30K (or 18.6 miles) gives you the feeling of a hard run like the half marathon but echoes the portion of the marathon where your glycogen stores begin to deplete and you need to call on mental strength[102]. Even the traditional 20-mile training runs don't simulate this energy output the way a 30K race does. So now that I have sold you on the idea of this distance, you might as well race the one which is "Older than Boston." That's right, one year older than the Boston Marathon, this race is also perfectly situated in the calendar for many to get their last long run in before Boston itself.

But if it were just the distance, that could be done anywhere. Around the Bay showcases some extraordinarily beautiful homes in Hamilton, while punishing you on a series of hills throughout the latter half. Big hills later in the race. *scratches chin thoughtfully* Where have I heard that before? *cough* BOSTON *cough*

The race has a later start in the day with the gun firing at 9:30 a.m. For us night owls, that is a wonderful time to start. Plenty of time to wake, eat, and vacate anything you may need to vacate.

---

[102] Or whatever deity you pray to when you need things. You never just call to say hello, do you?

Run This Place

It is also almost the same exact time of the day of that little ole marathon in Beantown.[103]

The course begins at the Ontario Dome before heading into a part of the race which was first added in 2014. Even though the distance didn't change, long-time runners say this addition adds a good minute to their overall time.[104] Through the city's gritty industrial district, this portion is hardly scenic. It also tends to be a tad spectator-sparse and highly exposed to the elements. Fortunately, you only encounter this dearth of cheering at the beginning of the race. To be quite honest, if you need cheers here, well, you might be in for a long day.

There are several overpasses you must traverse which give you just the right amount of muscle-use- differential[105] to keep you awake and ready for the remainder of the race. An early challenge to test your mettle, so to speak.

As gritty as the first 10K is with regards to scenery, the remainder of the race is inversely charming. As mentioned, this second half of the race is where the worst of the hills are located. In fact, after a two-year hiatus, the signature hill, re-routed around because of construction, returned in 2017. Right next to Hamilton Cemetery, the quarter mile beast of Valley Inn Hill will greet you with two miles to go. Also there to greet you is the Grim Reaper himself. Fortunately, he just hands out high fives.[106] Finishing inside a dome is a little tricky with a couple of tight turns but you will appreciate the warmth in case it is cold outside. And it's Canada so that probably is going to be the case.

My favorite part of this entire race is how your finish time determines the color of medal you receive. In an era where bling is all the rage and some feel there is no difference between all the runners, it is still satisfying to award those who work a little harder.

---

[103] Man, both these races should be paying me for this.
[104] It couldn't possibly be the fact they are just older and slower, right?
[105] A term I am coining for my next book so I can claim I know a "new" way to run.
[106] Seriously, some guy dressed as Death stands in the middle of the street. Runners are weird.

My Experience:

As you read earlier in the book, I ran this race the day after doing the Cooper River Bridge Run in Charleston, SC. So after a race there, two flights to get me to Buffalo, a drive to Hamilton, Ontario and then staying with a friend[107], I was not ready for anything groundbreaking with regards to a finishing time.

I mentioned the less-than beautiful first portion of the race but I was in heaven as I just enjoyed stretching out my legs from the race the day beforehand. In fact, even dealing with the overpasses, by the time I hit the first 10K I was only twelve seconds slower at that point than I had been for the 10K the day before.

Every kilometer was marked with an inspirational quote or saying. This was an appreciated touch, especially when the crowds were a bit thinner. Given there are more kilometers than miles in 30K, you also get a bunch of signs to read. I saw one right around the half-way point which said:

"You can learn everything about yourself by running a 30K."

I turned to the group of guys next to me, nodded at the sign and said "What if I am not *that* curious? Can I just stop at 20K?" The muffled laughter made me feel a little better about myself and jolted me out of small slump I was experiencing. Passing over a grated drawbridge helped my energy even more. I absolutely love bridges. You may have heard.

When I hit that halfway point, I saw if I repeated the time for the second half I would run 2:05:02 for the race. That time would have pleased me. So I settled down and concentrated on making that happen. Granted, on numerous occasions I have run a marathon distance at a much faster pace than what was necessary to maintain my desired goal but today this pace would be stellar. Accepting where you are right now and not being too discouraged about it is the key to getting through running.[108]

---

[107] Who I learned after getting there had cats, to which I am unfortunately allergic. But who needs to breathe?
[108] Or life, really.

Soon thereafter began the series of tough hills which my wonderful host for the weekend had downplayed quite effectively. While I have no intention of making a mountain out of a molehill, I also don't want to pretend these weren't tough. In fact, I was forced on an occasion or two to walk for a short distance. It is always amazing how much those little breaks can recharge your engine and get you right back on the heels of those who just left you behind.

Unfortunately, while the hills were now behind me, the wind was not. A stiff breeze which had swirled a bit earlier in the race, and had been blocked some by those very same hills I cursed, was now full on in our faces as I turned to head home. A group of guys numbering at least twelve went by me working together. I fell into this pack knowing I did not wish to fight the wind alone. But their pace was too quick. An internal debate waged on inside me as to whether I wanted to slow down and fight the wind alone or continue to run harder than I had in me in order to stay sheltered. I decided too late to ease off the throttle and when I finally slowed my pace, I came to yet another walk. Bollocks.

As I geared up running again, I heard some in the crowd mention the 2:10 pacer was coming up behind me. Double bollocks. I didn't really expect to be pushing hard to stay in front of him with 4K to go. Nonetheless, he soon passed me with another group of guys. Like before I fell in behind them. Unlike before their pace was more manageable.

For the next mile or so I hung tight until the group started to break up. Some fell off the back; others smelled the barn and began pushing for home. As I had started the race behind the 2:10 guy I knew I had some time to spare to make that time. As such, if I kept up, I should have no problem breaking 2:10. Hitting the 29K mark I had exactly five minutes to go under the desired goal time. I knew that even a slow kilometer was 4:30 and with this downhill finish, I might actually push hard and salvage a 2:08:59.

As the stadium came into view I noticed I couldn't see where the runners entered for the indoor finish. I looked at my watch and realized this was going to be much closer than it should be. Finally, I saw runners turning and heading down a Zamboni ramp[109]. A clock outside the stadium showed me I had only 25 seconds to break 2:10. I gritted my teeth, made the turn down the tunnel, and was immediately made blind by the change from bright sunshine to indoor darkness. At the bottom of this double-tiered ramp with a flat section in the middle, we had to make another quick 90-degree turn onto the field. I felt I probably had no chance to break 2:10.

I gave it everything I had in the final yards and hit my watch well after the finish. It showed 2:10:02. I knew I had some leeway from the chiptime but I didn't know how much. When I finally got the official results I found out it wasn't enough. My time was 2:10:00.4. Drats. Given I have never run a 30K, my positive spin was this was an instant PR. Or, since we were in the Great White North, a PB.[110] I finished 268th out of 7,277 finishers for one of my worst percentage-wise finishes in quite some time.

A bunch of Canadians owe me an "I'm sorry."

---

[109] It probably had nothing to do with a Zamboni but give this to me, ok?
[110] They call it a "personal best" here in Canada, eh.

Race: Fox Valley 20

Typical Date: Third Sunday in September

Distance: 20 miles

Location: St. Charles, IL

Why You Should Run It:

There are very few 20-mile races out there. Like the 30K whose virtues I extoll, the 20-mile distance is also excellent for those looking to make the leap from half marathon to marathon. Now just any 20-miler will suffice for training purposes but you need more than that to make it into this book, mister.[111] Running along the banks of the Fox River on flat, shaded bike paths is an ideal way to take on this distance and one way to help make this race a must-run. Moreover, set smack in the middle of September, with your fall marathon getting closer, this race is an absolutely perfect substitute for that last long training run you might have been dreading.

My Experience:

All three races of the weekend (marathon, half and 20-miler) are run on the same course which consists quite frequently of a narrow bike path. As such, the race organizers wisely send out runners in waves separated by fifteen seconds each in order to minimize congestion on the path. I had met the race director's daughter, Shannon, before the race and she was hoping to run a fast marathon. I told her I would be happy to keep her company until our course split if she wanted me to help keep her on pace. Always in good spirits, she said she would be glad to have someone with her. It was her fifth marathon and she looked absolutely at ease, relaxed, and ready to rock it. I could see my only real goal was to not get in the way of her training and keep her on exact pace.

---

[111] Do not sass talk me. I will turn this book around right now.

As the miles ticked by, the weather got a little sloppier. Rain started to come down but it was far better than a hot and humid day. There were plenty of twists and turns, and river crossings, and loops and reverse loops. But at every turn there were volunteers directing runners in the right direction. Given all the different runners running different distances, this could have been a convoluted logistical mess. The race director in me was already marveling at how well things were going. Volunteers were fervently checking bibs to know where to direct people and vocalized that direction loudly.

There did not seem to be many true spectators out on the course. As we abutted a plethora of backyards and front yards, I wished this had been different. I always hope spectators in similar situations will come out to cheer on runners. Being able to walk out of your door and see, for free, the human struggle in an event where elites and average Joes compete against all obstacles seems to be too wonderful to pass up. But many do just that. At one point, while admiring the homes along the river, we saw some couples sitting in their living rooms, mere feet away from us, watching TV. I said we needed some pebbles to throw at their windows so they could at least turn around.

Around the fifth mile I heard some footsteps and we were soon joined by a runner who I had met at the expo the day before. Running the half marathon, she looked in great shape and I commented on how I thought she might be the first female. About a mile later, we crossed the Fox River again and she turned off for home. I found out later that not only did she set a new personal record a few miles later but at the age of 49, Angie won the entire race! Way to go, Angie!

Shannon and I continued onward crossing bridges and making loops and she looked like she was out for a jog. I was beginning to wonder if I was holding her back too much and whether we should both pick it up. But I told her we would get through the first ten miles at 3:10 pace exactly and I was not going to start deviating from the plan at this point.

We soon began the longest stretch of straight running for the entire race that we had yet to encounter. It allowed us to settle into a groove and just feel how things were going. Even when the rain intensified, for the most part we were sheltered by a vast array of trees and foliage.

We soon entered North Aurora, the tenth mile, and what would be my final few steps with Shannon. I told her to stick to the game plan and slowly close the gap on the pace group which was about 30 seconds ahead of us. I said they had been running fairly consistently the past few miles so she could rely on them to hold the correct pace. After about mile 16, she should, if she felt good, begin to start to quicken her pace. I really felt like I was telling someone something they didn't need to know and for the most part kept my yapper shut. Not long after, Shannon continued on the path and I made a turn to head back home. I bid her adieu and listened as she headed into an aid station which echoed with cheers.

The second half of my race was quite uneventful and in a long-distance race that is a good thing. From the split around mile 10.5 to mile 14, the course was quite lonely. Actually, while the runners were alone I wouldn't say I was lonely. In fact, this time was a chance to look inward and see how the body was feeling. I was hoping to run about 30 seconds faster per mile for the second half of this race but for the most part I could see that was not happening. So while I would pick off the occasional racer ahead of me, I spent those miles thinking about, well, sometimes everything and sometimes nothing.

At mile 14, the course rejoined the half marathon course and now I had more people to try to encourage. I had no idea whatsoever what place I was in with regards to my race and I did not care. I was taking in the splendor of the course and the shared spirit of all those out here working their butts off.

Around the 16th mile I passed the lead female and offered her some words of encouragement. She looked like she might be having a rough day but I knew there was no one close to her. It was here where I realized that if my math was right and my pace was true, I could possibly run a 2:22:22. I love stuff like this. It is quirky little number games I play with myself in races that aren't actually "races" in order to keep me interested and fresh. So with each mile I passed I tried to see how much I had to speed up or slow down in order to accomplish this task. Passing runners was fun but it was not what I was thinking of doing as the miles ticked by. I did see another runner in front of me and while I was closing the gap with each mile, I figured I would really have to haul over the last two miles to pass him. I saw no reason to do so. First, I had no idea what place we were fighting for. Second, this was meant to be a training run for me and I needed to keep it as such.[112]

Nearing the end, I could see I was running too fast for the 2:22:22. I would have had to come to a dead stop to get that time and that is just a little silly. So I cruised through the finish in 2:22:14, enjoying a sixth place overall finish and my first ever 20-mile race.

---

[112] To be completely truthful, if I had known the guy in front of me was fifth place, I might have picked it up a little bit. I mean, it is the top five.

Race: San Felipe Shootout

Typical Date: Fourth Saturday in March

Distance: 5K, 10K, and Half marathon-ish

Location: Stephen F. Austin State Park, San Felipe, TX

Why You Should Run It:

Experiencing a race like this which is really three different races but also sorta kinda one race all wrapped into one is an experience unto itself.

The course is mostly a single track hiking/biking trail in San Felipe State Park. A fairly flat race except for a few dips to small creeks and some elevation change around the Brazos River, it has the luxury of being a trail race that is still quite runnable. The course itself is primarily under a forest canopy which will help keep the sun at bay. The 5K is one loop, 10K is the 5K route twice, and the half marathon was three loops of the 5K course with a few added out-and-backs.

The order of events for the day is to start with the 5K first, followed by the 10K an hour later, and then the half marathon two hours after the 10K. The faster you finish each race, the more rest you have. The winner is determined by the person with the lowest combined time of all three races. As such, runners are presented with the battle of figuring out how much energy they should expend on each race, with three races' efforts cut up with breaks. This is truly a unique and exciting way to run nearly a marathon distance over the course of a morning.

My Experience:

Out of the gate, we ran out of the parking lot and plunged into the trail. The soft forgiving dirt was pleasantly runnable, but the path was hardly smooth or straight. We ran counterclockwise, with two out-and-backs allowing us to see many, but not all, of the participants behind us. We were lucky this year to have dry footing as the previous two years had been mucky and "possessing of moats", one person told me.[113]

I started out in about sixth or seventh place, not pushing too hard knowing that a 5K is not my type of race, a trail is not my type of footing, and I did not know the course as many running already did. Today's effort was not about doing well in a sprint 5K but rather doing well overall in the combined races. Unfortunately, even running relatively conservatively, I found myself unable to breathe, a problem I had been dealing with going into the race for the previous week. For the entirety of the 5K I was nearly clutching at my chest, waiting for the body to realize it was racing, and clear up the passages. It never happened.

In spite of my breathing-through-a-straw strategy, I still came into the finish in 13th place overall. I peeled off my shirt and wrung out about three pounds of sweat. Rob Goyen, the RD and one heck of a guy, stared as the river of sweat poured off of me. I toweled off, put on a different shirt, drank a ton of fluids, and got ready for the 10K to start in 35 minutes.

I had debated carrying my handheld Camelbak bottle for the 10K but figured that even though the only aid station was at the end of the loop, and you would have to go a few feet out of your way to get it, I would simply go without. I took a big ole swig of water before the start of the race and got ready to rock. I figured I was now fully awake, had coughed out the crap in my lungs for the 5K, and would be ready to turn on the jets. Ready! Aim!

Millennium Falcon HyperDrive Fail Noise

There was absolutely no response from my body at all. No kick in the legs and definitely no air from the lungs. As we made our first out-and-back, I was wondering what the rest of the day would hold. Then as I was making a turn, I saw some runners coming back

---

[113] Dibs on "Possessing of Moats" for the name of a band.

toward me when they weren't supposed to be. They passed me and I asked the trailing runner what was happening. Apparently, a runner or two went the wrong way and these people were backtracking thinking they were going the wrong way. I came to a stop, grabbed one runner, and yelled at the rest, "It is a 5K loop we run twice. Come back here!" When I saw that the runners in sight were heading back, I continued on my way. I think every one of the runners I yelled at passed me within seconds. Even with a head start, I couldn't perform.[114]

Resigned to run out the loop, I just put my head down and trudged onward. In this state of acquiescence I moved through the forest and was more than pleased to see the end of the loop in sight. As I turned around the cone and headed out for the second loop, I was surprised that I wasn't all that much slower in this first 5K of the 10K then I was in the 5K itself. Typical Dane: no impressive top speed but I can hold it forever.

My goal for this loop was to simply keep as many people behind me as possible. For the next mile I just sort of hung in place. Suddenly, at the infamous "Touch me and Turn Around" sign, it was like someone put a siphon into my lungs and sucked all the crap out of them. Feeling like a new runner, I went from 7:30 miles to 6:30 with ease.

There were just two more guys for me to try to pass as we neared the end. Almost in their back pocket I felt the slightest twinge of a cramp. Knowing I had 13.1 more miles to go, and sprinting here was pointless, I slowed a touch in the last quarter mile, still negative-splitting the race. My place was 17th overall which was hardly what I had wanted but far better than what it could have been if I had continued my lethargic slide.

But then I sat down.

For the next hour I fought with myself about whether I even wanted to run the half marathon. The day was already not going where I had wanted it to go. As the heat continued to rise, I knew

---

[114] That's what she said.

my chances of performing better were lessening greatly. A friend told me she had never seen me look so utterly crestfallen before in a race.

I tried to figure out if I should go on. I finally decided that my original intention was to use this day of racing as a prep run for a 50K coming up in a month. If I was going to get a proper day of training in, it wasn't going to be by running 9.5 miles. So, I finally sucked it up and decided that yes, I would run, but it would just be slow. No longer would I care about who I beat but instead today would be about smartly running the remaining miles.

When the half started it was now in the high 70s but the humidity had at least dropped. I donned my Camelbak backpack and thanked the running gods I had the foresight to freeze the bladder beforehand. Half ice-water now because of the heat, it barely registered cold on my back as I slid it on.

As we began the first loop, I hung tight to the right side of the trail letting anyone who wanted to pass me, do so. Not many did but I was obviously not in the position I had been in previous races on the day. During this first loop, I can honestly say that I could not have cared less about finishing the half marathon. I can count on one hand the number of times in a race where I felt as abjectly disheartened as I did here. I did my best to not think. Left, right, repeat. It didn't improve.

While the whole loop is trail, there was one section that suited me better than any other. A completely flat, straight section with no twisting or turning presented itself in front of me with footing as soft as you can hope for on a trail. Each time I hit this part I would pick up the pace and close gaps on runners. Closing in on the first loop, I passed a few runners and began feeling decent. As I started the next loop, I thought perhaps I would finish after all.

This half marathon loop was marginally different than the other loops in order to make the distance as accurate as possible. There was a small dogleg section halfway through the loop where we ran through a mostly dry river bed. The previous year this area had chest-deep water from some torrential rain earlier in the season. I wondered if I would sacrifice the potential chafing for some cooling wetness here but then remembered how bad I chafe from my own sweat and decided against that.

As my pace picked up near the end of this second loop, I could see I was in the top ten. However, on the straight stretch I mentioned above, I felt a slight twinge in my hamstrings again. I knew at some point the dehydration would have an effect but I didn't know when that would be. I approached the end of the loop and decided that while stopping short was hardly what I wanted to do, it was the wise move. I went through the end of the loop, stopped my watch and sat down. I was done.

Drinking heavily from some ice cold beverages, I grabbed a towel and wiped myself dry. I continued to sit there for about ten minutes or so. I then decided to go to the bathroom. To my surprise, there weren't any signs of massive dehydration like I would have expected. I drank a little bit more and dunked my head in an ice bucket. Talking to Rob again, he told me there wasn't a darn thing wrong with stopping but I could take all the time in the world to finish if I wanted to. He again commented on the deluge of sweat which cascaded off of me. I figured I might as well give the rest of the race a shot.

Out I went again on the third loop, after close to 20 minutes of downtime. To my surprise, my legs were not nearly as cramped or stiff as I assumed they would be. I began passing runners left and right and feeling far better than I had any right to feel. Obviously well behind where I should have been, the break, toweling, and ice had obviously combated some of the worse effects of the heat and my own DNA. The loop went by rather uneventfully and I found myself back at the start. While I did not sit down for 20 minutes again, I did take another break, sat for a bit, toweled off again, and jammed a chunk of ice between my CamelBak and my back. Now with only three miles to go, I knew I would at least finish. My time was of no concern.

Because of that knowledge, I spent the first .6 of a mile in a fast walk. I wanted to go faster but people in Hell want ice water. So I went with what I knew would work and that was measured forward motion. Finally, feeling well enough to run, I took off. As I passed some of the same people for like the third time in less time than it should take to pass someone three times (they had all passed me on one of my breaks) one guy in a huge sombrero asked "How many laps are you doing?!" I told him I decided to quit. Then decided I was bad at quitting and began again. He cheered me on and I gave him a thumbs up.[115]

I may have passed another runner or two near the finish but it was of no matter. I crossed the finish line in 39th place overall and could not have been more tickled to be done. I also was beyond proud of myself for not only persevering but doing so wisely. If I had put my health or the overall objective to prepare for this 50K in jeopardy, I would have stopped. But by running smart, I finished.

All told, out of 107 people who finished the Triple race, I was 18th overall. Take out just the 20-minute break and I would have been in the top ten. However, without that break who knows if I would have even finished. Without a doubt the day did not turn out as planned. With running, pushing your body to perform, that happens. The bad days far outweigh the good days. You just hope the good days fall on race day.

---

[115] It is entirely possible he was a hallucination.

Marathons

Race: First Light Marathon

Typical Date: Second Sunday in January

Distance: Marathon

Location: Mobile, AL

Why You Should Run It:

The First Light Marathon is put on by the Mobile, Alabama branch of a group called L'Arche. An International Federation, L' Arche (French for "The Ark", as in "Noah's Ark") is dedicated to the creation and growth of homes, programs, and support networks for people with intellectual disabilities. Races having a charitable component are almost a no-brainer these days. This race has more than a tenuous connection as it goes hand-in-hand with the L'Arche organization itself. Residents of L'Arche's home not only create all the finisher medals and age group awards but are on-hand at the finish to personally hand them to every runner as well.

The marathon streams along the mossy tree-lined streets of Mobile, through the campuses of the University of South Alabama and Spring Hill College, before finishing in the beautiful and historic Bienville Square, named for the founder of Mobile. Belles in full historic dress with twirling parasols greet you along the way with buttery-thick accents and ringlets in their hair. Weather-wise, one would be hard pressed to pick a better time to race in Mobile than in January. Even though you may get a warm day with a bit of mugginess, chances are high you would have a fine day for racing.

Mobile itself is an amazing city which was struck hard by Hurricane Katrina. Often overlooked because of the damage that New Orleans sustained, the area here had a tough go getting itself back on its feet. Now, over a decade later, it is thriving again and there are few places which exude southern charm more than the Azalea City.

The course is forgiving with just a touch of hills here and there.

OK, there is a tough steady climb around mile eleven but that is far enough into the race that you should be warmed up by then. You'll encounter a quick up and down before entering the University, where cheerleaders are out to boost your spirits. Finally, right at mile eighteen, you have your last hill of the day before a great downhill with a 10K to go. After that it is a long, flat stretch with just two quick turns for you to focus on your finish line smile.

My Experience:

In the interest of full disclosure, it would be nearly impossible for me not to include this race in this book if only for personal reasons. When I ran my 52 marathons in 52 weekends in 2006, this particular branch of L'Arche in Mobile was the beneficiary of all the funds I raised during the year. When I was planning my endeavor the year prior, I happened upon this race. I inquired more about for whom they were working, and was taken aback. I had worked with mentally and physically challenged people in a multitude of ways since I was quite young. For me not to have even heard of this organization meant many others who had not been involved so intimately were undoubtedly just as much in the dark about its existence. As such, I took it upon myself to not only raise money[116] but to spread the word about them far and wide. When I ran the race I could not have been more pleased with how well organized it was. The fact it was also benefitting people I truly cared about was just icing on the cake. I ran it again in 2010 on an inexplicably cold day when I ran back-to-back marathons in Jackson, Mississippi and there. These two races remain the only two marathons in which I have ever worn full tights. Even for me, fourteen degrees is too cold to just wear shorts.[117]

The overall feel of this race is one of unpretentiousness but also competence. The organizers' laidback nature belies their intricate planning and attention to detail. With the race hotel being literally feet away from the start and half a mile from the finish, logistics-wise this is a huge plus. Wake up, walk outside, run, walk a few

---
[116] Over $43,000 when all was said and done.
[117] I may wish to sire children.

blocks back to your hotel, shower and be on your way.

Personally seeing the faces of those I was specifically helping with my fundraising was an amazing experience. Even if you raise money for a good cause, you are often far removed from those you are directly helping. Lost in the largeness of an organization, you know you are helping in some grander sense of things but your connection is tenuous at best. Here, I got to get to know people on a personal level and it made my entire 52 marathons that much more meaningful. It wasn't just about me completing the hardest thing I had ever done. It was about getting the word out about an organization that truly needed to be known. Having that added motivation kept me going through tough times and sore muscles. Even as the years have passed and some of the residents have left this earth, I think about them all and how much they helped me do something previously thought impossible.

The first year I ran this marathon is a little hazy for me to recall as it was just the second of the 52 I ran that year. Getting underway and knowing I still had 50 left means some of the finer details of that event are lost. That said, the year I ran in the cold is unforgettable. Racing back-to-back marathons was hard but the unexpected cold added another layer of difficulty, as well as a layer of clothes. After a relatively uneventful first half of the race where I was simply trying to get the muscles moving after a fast marathon the day before, I came upon a solo female runner. For the next seven miles, Anna and I ran together. This was only her third marathon and she had never run this particular race before. As such, I started to provide helpful tips here and there, assisting where I could. I gave sage advice on how to pace, where to surge in the race depending on the terrain, and how to effectively utilize my vast knowledge to help her succeed.

Then we made a wrong turn because I am the best guide ever.

A friend of mine also running the race saw us make the mistaken turn. When he got to that intersection, he yelled at the top of his lungs. Fortunately we heard him and turned around before going too far. No idea to this day why we made that wrong turn there as it was clearly marked. Catching my friend, we thanked him

Run This Place

profusely and then blazed on by. With about a 10K to go, I could tell she was ready to leave me behind. I mentioned I thought there was only one woman in front of us and I hope she caught her.

She did.

I spent the last few miles trying to adhere to a strict pace. You see, I had decided before the race that I was going to run a 3:17. With this being my 110th marathon, it was not as if the luster of racing the distance had disappeared but it was a welcome change to spruce things up once in a while. So, being a bit of a geeky numbers guy, I decided to run a 3:17 as I had never run that specific time. I had run numerous 3:16s and a 3:18 (and almost every single other time from 2:55 to 3:30) but not that number in between. So, no matter how good or bad I felt throughout the race, I did everything I could to run between 7:30 to 7:33 per mile as that would bring me in somewhere in the minute of 3:17. This may sound easy but it way harder than one might think. Often, as you near the end of the race, you pick up the pace as you can visualize the finish. But here, no matter what, I just had to keep an even keel.

Along the last stretch of miles I ran alone, Anna having disappeared into the horizon. I passed the only other female in front of me and was in a bit of a zone. With about a quarter of a mile to go, I could see that I was going to finish right smack dab in the middle of the 3:17 minute. Suddenly three guys sprinted past me and began their own battle for a finishing place. One of the things I wish we could do is plug into each person's mind as they run to see what their goals were for the day. What was motivating them. Why they were surging. What time they were hoping to hit. Whether this finish was going to disappoint or elate them.

As I had nothing to gain by countering their sprint and couldn't care less about where I finished, I blissfully allowed them to sail by without a care in the world. I finished in 3:17:37 and found out these last three guys had pushed me out of the top 20.

You dirty no-good S.O.B.s.[118]

---

[118] I am kidding. Mostly.

Dane Rauschenberg

Race: Kiawah Island Marathon

Typical Date: Second Saturday in December

Distance: Marathon

Location: Kiawah Island, SC

Why You Should Run It:

With the proliferation of marathons, it is hard to find a race which has which really throws its all into celebrating its runners. While the Kiawah Island Marathon is held on a luxury golf resort, virtually everyone you run into on the island is either running the race, cheering the race, or impressed that you are running the race. Furthermore, as the island is rather secluded from the mainland, you don't necessarily run into too many people anyway. You feel isolated but in a good way. Away from the troubles and thoughts of the outside world.

The course itself enjoys spectacular views of maritime forests, marshes, and grand homes, as you run throughout the island community. One of the flattest marathons out there, the elevation chart looks horrendous until you realize the big hill at the beginning and end climbs eight feet (2.4 meters).[119] While the exact configuration of the course has changed since I ran it twice, it remains similar. My two runnings in 2010 and 2011 were two loops of the same half course. Some like that; some don't. The reason I prefer a course of this nature is that the surprise is taken out of what lies ahead.

For the next three years after I last ran Kiawah there were a ton of U-turns and sidewalk running as they tested out some new courses. However, in 2016 the organizers seemed to find a course that eliminates the worst of everything and really allows runners to run. You may, as a faster marathon, run into slower half marathoners walking three-abreast on narrower paths but

---
[119] I am kidding. Who doesn't know what eight feet is?

Run This Place

not every race is perfect.

The twisting nature of the course affords your well-wishers the ability to easily get around to a variety of spots on a bicycle (or on foot) to cheer you on. It will take a bit of planning, and maybe a map, but seeing loved ones often throughout a race, instead of only at the beginning and the end, provides oodles of gumption on race day.

This is not a race for those who need tons of people to cheer them on. As I mentioned, it is on an island that is almost entirely inhabited by those playing golf. But that slight isolation allows you the opportunity to be worry-free about street closures, errant vehicles, or all the trappings which come with bigger races.

Weather in South Carolina in December is almost always pleasant for racing. Rarely do you get a warm day even if it may still be a bit humid. As the year closes down, it is hard to find a better weather day for a race across the country. For my money, good weather beats out a good course.

What I really like about this race is that it is held on a Saturday. The vast majority of runners make a weekend out of it and stay around after the race for another day. It is one thing to mingle with runners before a race; it is an entirely separate thing to do so the day after. When the goal has been accomplished and you can simply reminisce on what happened, good or bad, it is altogether pleasant.

My Experience:

I have run both the marathon and the half marathon at Kiawah. When I ran the marathon I was recovering from strep throat. When I ran the half I was coming off of an Achilles injury. In spite of these ailments, I had an enjoyable race in which I ran respectable times. Says a great deal about the event itself if you can come into it lame and still enjoy the outcome.[120]

When I ran the marathon, it was my 16th of that year and I finished

---
[120] Or your insanity level.

in 3:05:41 in some rainy conditions. What is intriguing about this finish time is I had previously run another 3:05:41 marathon. The first time I had done so was at the Erie Marathon at Presque isle in 2007. The Erie Marathon is also a two-loop course, on an almost pancake flat surface, which I also ran in a heavy rain. Erie's race, also on essentially what is an island[121], has limited traffic on the course, and is surrounded by lush trees for the entirety of the race. In addition the races were started just three years apart (1974 for Erie and 1977 for Kiawah).[122]

With the half marathon I ran, I had an extremely odd experience. Right around the tenth mile of a relatively uneventful race, a small group of runners who had been catching me passed me by. A slight woman, who looked strangely familiar, cut in front of me. Her action did not necessarily trip me but it definitely made me do a small stutter step. It did put me a little off though as there was no real need for her to cut that quickly in front of me right there. Granted, if the woman was running the half, she was fighting for one of the top five spots overall but it wasn't as if we were setting the course ablaze back here in 1:23-1:25 land. After dropping back for a second, I decided that I did not want to be running behind her anymore. Just one of those "Nah, that's not how this is going to play" reactions. So I surged again, getting energy out of nowhere and soon was a few yards in front of the group. Here I would stay for a few miles, until a game of cat and mouse with a series of runners would have us all changing places.

When the race was finished I was looking over the results. I saw the small woman had not been running the half but had instead been running the marathon. Without a doubt that made her effort in the first half all the more impressive. While her second half showed a large slowing down (ten minutes slower than her first half) what stood out was her name: Zola Pieterse. That might

---

[121] Presque Isle is a peninsula with just a .15-mile swatch of land in width connecting it to the mainland.

[122] To be honest, I quit researching their similarities as I thought I might unravel the spacetime continuum and then there is just no way you will be able to get to run all these races. You are welcome.

not immediately ring a bell for you but if we went by her maiden name perhaps you would understand the surrealness of my situation. You see, the woman who almost tripped me was none other than Zola Budd – the diminutive runner who was involved in an unfortunate incident in the 1984 Olympics where her feet tangled with American sweetheart runner Mary Decker Slaney. When I realized I had almost repeated history with Mrs. Pieterse my mouth dropped wide open. Only in the sport of running can something like this happen.

I finished the half marathon in 1:25:11, good enough for 41st place overall in my 52nd lifetime half marathon. Of those 52 races, 31 had been run during the previous a year and a half. In fact, when I finished my 100th lifetime marathon in 2009 I had only run 14 half marathons. Now I was well on my way to 100 half marathons.

So, run Kiawah and Zola Budd might trip you is the moral of the story.

Dane Rauschenberg

Race: Run with the Horses

Typical Date: Third Saturday in August

Distance: Marathon

Location: Green River, WY

Why You Should Run It:

Many races promise a variety of different amenities and views of famous sites. As you will learn by participating in enough of them, even a large building goes by pretty quickly when you are running. And as much as I like running on bridges, the views of a bridge are often far more pretty when taken from a great distance away. In other words, the main draw of scenic races is often for everyone but the actual runners. Having said that, where else will you get a chance to run amongst herds of wild horses at the top of a high desert plateau?

You will have to work for your view as you start at roughly 6,100 feet before climbing 1,400 feet in nine miles. But once you are up in the rarefied air, the Old West feeling comes out. Do not run this race if you need tons of cheering crowds. You will not find them. You might not find any people whatsoever, except for the volunteers strategically placed every two miles at the aid stations. All told there may be a collective total of 100 runners in all the races. As the race is run in a high desert, you can expect a very dry climate. There is not one single ounce of shade on the course so whatever Mother Nature decides to give you, you will get.

Now, I just listed a variety of things that will make some people tap out immediately. But I know just as many are salivating at the thought of taking on so many challenges. To be quite honest, once you have crested the highest point and have the opportunity to look out over the whole valley, all of your effort feels justified.

As for the namesake of this race, your own experience with seeing horses will vary as they are, as mentioned, wild. But many have reported seeing golden eagles and pronghorn to go along with the horses, as well. Running here on the plains is as if you are getting your own Where the Buffalo Roam song being played out in front of your eyes. The best part of the course may be the finish where you get to go back down that long hill you had to climb in the beginning. Save your legs for the descent!

My Experience:

I ran this race with a heavy heart in honor of a friend who had unexpectedly passed away just a few days prior. I wanted to win the race for him but in reality I wanted to think about anything other than the frailty of life. The course is slightly different now than when I ran it as we had a point-to-point but the final 13.1 miles are the same. Unfortunately, it was before I even got to the starting line that I experienced some problems.

The year I ran the race there were only two Porta-Potties at the start, which you think would be enough. You would be wrong.[123] It appeared every single person in front of me was performing a 16-step routine in the bathroom. The average time was two minutes and forty-five seconds per person.[124] What the heck were they doing?

As the clock wound down to the 6:30 a.m. start, I was assured they would hold the start for a few minutes, as it was clear there were many still in line to use the loo. However, with three separate races starting on the same clock, I knew there would be no waiting. As it was such a small race, there was also no chip-timing, so, when the runners started and I was still one person away from the bathroom, I was SOL[125]. Unfortunately, what I needed to do, NEEDED to be done here. I finally got into the toilet and did the fastest "business" you could possibly imagine. By the time I got out, I figured I was already a good two minutes behind. If you check your latest "How to Run a Smart Race" in Runner's

---

[123] General rule of thumb: quintuple the number of participants and that is still not enough bathrooms. I am kidding. Slightly.
[124] Yep, I was timing them.
[125] No, MST3K fans, this is not "Satellite of Love."

World, this is not listed anywhere in the checklist.

After a few miles of catch-up running I was third place. In hindsight, I knew I should not have tried to make up all the lost time so quickly. When I slipped into this position, I could see the other two runners were ahead of me by just about the amount of time I had spent in the bathroom. This weighed far more heavily on my mind than it should have. There was no controlling it and I should have put it to rest earlier than I did. Fortunately, the surrounding scenery finally got my mind on something else.

The high plains were a stark contrast to the forest I grew up with in Pennsylvania. Heck, they were even different than the mountains I lived next to in Salt Lake City at the time. One might be tempted to say there was a lot of "nothing." Doing so is a lazy way to describe a vast plain, set 7,500 feet above sea level. It was open. It was rather uninterrupted. But it was far from nothing. Then I saw them.

I would like to claim that a pack of wild horses encircled me, kicking up dust, and wedded me in oneness with my equine brethren. That did not happen. Nevertheless, more than a dozen horses appeared to my right, manes flapping in the wind, and trotting along at an easy pace. They looked a little unkempt and well, wild. For more than a few minutes I was lost watching them. Wondering how close they would come, I forgot about my own race for a bit. They never got closer than fifty yards or so but others spoke open-mouthed about being almost within touching distance. Horses are so commonplace for some people, their size and strength is sometimes forgotten.[126] Here I was able to simply enjoy their company before they suddenly decided to go a different direction. I was horseless again like a person who had no horses.[127]

Well over the halfway point now, I felt I was closing in on the two guys in front of me. With no discernible features to gauge distance and time, I couldn't be sure but they appeared to be getting closer.

---
[126] I have often said that it would be absolutely terrifying if horses were carnivorous.
[127] I write the most beautiful similes.

The slight twisting nature of the course, with small rises up and down, would often allow those I was chasing to disappear from view. The miles slid by with me in pursuit.

Mile 21 went up and around a bend. At one point I could see the town of Green River in the distance to my left with a dirt road leading down to it. To the right was another dirt road which faced north and looked like it ran unimpeded until it hit Montana. As the two runners in front of me were nowhere to be found, I had little to go on in determining which path to take. I saw some red paint on the ground leading to the left. I figured this must be the way since the town was below it. So I took the road. I figured wrong.

After a good quarter of a mile, the road became very straight and I could see no other runner in front of me for miles. Crap. I took the wrong road. Back up the hill I went, thoroughly demoralized. I took the other fork and about five minutes later saw the mile 22 marker on my right. There had been some other paint on the ground that I simply hadn't seen which told me to take the road to the right. I guess this is one of the "problems" with being at the front of the pack.

The final few miles were on a long downhill, through a canyon of sorts. I was trying desperately to make up time from the detour and bathroom break but still was taken back by the beauty. I remember saying out loud: "This is really pretty."

One feature which was almost laughable in its cruelty (and one you no longer have to deal with because of the course change) is a ramp up and over the main highway, followed by a set of stairs on the other side to get back down. I recalled reading that one of the first New York City Marathons had something similar where runners had to incorporate a stair workout into the final stretch of their race. If you think your legs are tired at the end of a marathon, throw in a few steps.

Finally, as I crossed the finish, my time was still a Boston Qualifier, but only by my watch. The official clock time had me running a 3:12 which ended a long streak of consecutive BQs. Streaks come to an end and that is always unfortunate. But if it had to do happen somewhere, running with wild horses seemed like a great place for it.

Run This Place

Race: Boston Marathon

Typical Date: Patriot's Day

Distance: Marathon

Why You Should Run It:

Just because some races are often listed as a must-do does not mean they shouldn't be included in every list. And the Boston Marathon is indeed a race that should be on every single person's radar. Entire libraries of tomes have been written about the lore and love of Boston. Since the bombings in 2013, it has become even more historic, more prestigious, and more a part of the running journey for so many runners. Sure, it is a bit of a logistical pain in the butt. But it is one of the few races out there, nay one of the few things in life, which in spite of the hype and pomp and circumstance, somehow surpasses expectations.

My Experience

I have run Boston officially twice: 2005 and 2008. However, in 2008, I ran it another unofficial time. Dave McGillivray, who has been the race director for many years, has a tradition of running the race after it is all underway and his immediate attention can be delegated away from his well-oiled machine. He runs this post-race marathon to keep his streak of running the Boston Marathon alive. I had assisted Dave on an event back in 2007 where we became acquaintances and I had learned about his amazing running story. When 2008 rolled around, I asked if he would mind if I joined him on his run.

Simply running 52.4 miles in one day is a challenge but after running a 3:01 for the first official marathon, I had a rather unenviable task afterward. First, I had to wade through the rigmarole of the end of the marathon. Then I had to make my way back too Dave's hotel. Unfortunately, he was not there and as I did not have a key, I couldn't even get into the hotel lobby. I was hoping for a quick shower, a change of clothes, and maybe a bite to eat before heading back out to Hopkinton to do it all over again. No such luck. After about 90 minutes of sitting on a cold sidewalk, Dave appeared out of nowhere and asked me if I was ready. He had obviously been tending to one of his thousand jobs that day and was ready to go get his run started. That meant no time for the things I was hoping to do. No food and no shower and then next thing I knew I was in a director's chair in the back of a van betwixt boxes of extra Boston Marathon jackets rollicking down the Mass Pike to the start.

When we finally got out of the van, I had just enough time to change shirts, reapply some lubricant, pour a bottle of water over my head as a makeshift shower and jam some Oreo cookies in my mouth. Let's just say I was a little creaky when we started. But I would not have traded this experience for anything as the juxtaposition of running amongst hundreds of thousands of screaming fans a few hours earlier and the empty streets later was both surreal and priceless. I touched on the amazing experience I had near the end of the race in another one of my books so I won't repeat it here.

Just run Boston.

Race: Light at the End of the Tunnel Marathon/Tunnel Lite

Typical Date: Mid-July/Mid-September

Distance: Marathon

Location: North Bend, WA

Why You Should Run It:

The twice-named marathon is as such as it is one of the few events where the exact same course is run twice in a year.[128] The only

---

[128] In fact, it is so popular there has been infighting between these races and another from another company which wants to use the same exact course at a third time of year.

difference between the two is that the September race has fewer aid stations and is more of a BYOwhatever you need. However, both events feature two specifically wonderful things. The first is a gradually sloping downhill course which gives runners about eighty feet of grade per mile. While this can definitely be helpful, at no point does it feel like you are going to destroy your quads by running down some black diamond ski slope. Instead, it simply feels like you are having a good day.

The second aspect, and the namesake, is the over two-mile-long run in pitch black through an old railway tunnel. Entering from the east end, runners must wear headlights as they the traverse its length. The other end of the tunnel, which seems just a few hundred feet away, stays a pinprick of light for what feels like an unnaturally long period of time. Slowly and surely the light grows brighter, the tunnel opening grows larger, and eventually you can see the world on the other side.[129]

Once you leave the tunnel, you have a mostly crushed gravel course until about the twenty-first mile. After that you have a series of paved bicycle trails, followed once again by a hard-packed trail. The day can get a little warm in the July version, and with ever-increasingly warm summers thanks to this elaborate Chinese hoax of climate change, the September version is not guaranteed to be cool, either. Fortunately, the mostly shaded course allows runners to feel good for a very long period of time regardless of the temperature.

My Experience:

I have run both versions of this race and there is indeed something surreal and a little unsettling about running in a tunnel as long as Central Park in NYC. Popping out and handing your headlamp to a volunteer makes you feel like you have your own NASCAR pit crew. My two times running the race netted me results which were well in line with what I was hoping, including a 3:01 marathon in the July version. I had hoped for a sub-three to net a marathon starting with a "2" for the first time in the state of Washington but

---

[129] In other words, you can see the light at the... I am not even going to finish that.

as this was my third marathon in fourteen days, I would call it a success for sure.

When I ran it in September the next year, I was coming off what was my worst year of racing ever and was more than happy with the 3:06 I ran there.

Run This Place

Race: Deadwood Mickelson Trail Marathon

Typical Date: First Sunday in June

Distance: Marathon

Location: Deadwood, SD

Why You Should Run It:

The Deadwood Mickelson Trail Marathon is a point-to-point course[130], beginning in the hamlet of Rockford and ending at the historic Engine House near the Deadwood Trailhead. The first mile is paved, then the next 13 miles or so is a gradual uphill climb from about 5,500 feet to 6,200 feet. Once you hit that peak, the second half is mostly downhill. Run on a railroad trail on crushed gravel surface, it is both wide and forgiving to the feet. While a trail marathon for sure, it is one of the softest trails upon which you can run. But don't sleep on that elevation change or even the starting elevation point. Already higher than Denver and then going up 50 feet a mile for the first 13 miles, there is no point in which you think you are going up any major hill. But you will feel it in your lungs for sure.

The race is the brainchild of Jerry Dunn. Jerry made a name for himself by running 200 marathon distances in just one year. This included going to an actual marathon race, running on the day before and day after the race as well as the race itself. When I was researching my own 52 marathon journey in 2006 I came upon Jerry and we became friends. Hearing him speak so reverently about the race in the area where he lived, I knew I had to make it part of my 52.

Often a race's character is what separates it from others, especially in today's world where there are thousands of races each year. Don't get me wrong, the course is amazing. But when we think of

---

[130] A phrase I have always found interesting as every course is point-to-point, technically.

the Old West, there are basically two places which come to mind: Tombstone, Arizona and Deadwood, South Dakota. Once you step foot into the town you feel a shootout could break out at any moment (and it does with a daily re-enactment).

Unlike many trail races in serene settings where if you don't watch your footing you might end up tumbling into an abyss, the wide paths here allow you to take in every tunnel you barrel through, every stream crossing, and whatever wildlife which may cross your path.

My Experience:

When I took on this race in 2006 it was my first race as a 30-year-old. It was also just the second race I had run after getting braces on my teeth. I remember two things clearly; how beautiful everything around me appeared and how much my mouth hurt. Even though I finished 17th overall, I was still only fifth in my new age group. One week earlier in I would have been nipping on the heels of the guy who won my younger group. In fact, in a race where there were sometimes many minutes between each runner, here there were seven of us separated by just a shade over a minute. I remember that for the majority of the race I always had someone a few yards ahead of me, next to me or behind me. Furthermore, after I finished, two other fellas came barreling past the finish in the next sixteen seconds.

This was my 22nd marathon in as many weeks. The summer was beginning and I was quite beat. Somehow though the cool mountain air and crispness of non-humidity woke up a little racer in me. This was probably the highest elevation I had even been in my life until that point and definitely the highest marathon.[131] Nevertheless, I was able to run exceedingly well given all of the circumstances.

I also had an increasingly odd experience on race weekend which,

---

[131] Outside of a paragliding in the town of Zermatt Switzerland while in law school – and upon checking the elevation I am shocked to see that Deadwood is actually higher up than Zermatt. Could I leave all of this out and edit it? Sure. But I like you, the reader, to see the effort I go to for your enjoyment and accuracy.

looking back, seems like something I wonder why I ever did. To make a long story short, on the flight to Rapid City, which was the closest airport, I sat next to a gentleman who had some sort of physical ailment. He told me he was heading to Deadwood as he had been in an accident there sometime before as a pedestrian hit by a car. His return trip was being made to collect information or speak to a lawyer about adding crosswalks to the area in which he was hit.

I helped him with his things both on the airplane and at the luggage carousel. When he mentioned he was going to Deadwood and coming back the day I needed to head to the airport, he said he could save me some cash on a rental car. I readily accepted even though, in hindsight, this sounds like a horrific idea. The drive was over an hour away and if he just decided to ditch me at any point, I would have had no car and no way to get ahold of anyone. As I was funding my whole adventure out of my own pocket, I was always looking for ways to cut costs. It sometimes clouded my judgment.

Obviously, everything worked out fine. But this does seem like the sort of story that begins with Keith Morrison creepily discussing my severed head found in a roadside rest stop on Dateline NBC.[132]

---

[132] There was also some weird thing with a hotel room that I cannot for the life of me remember what went down but I ended up getting a crappy last-minute hotel, too. Seriously, I should probably be dead right now.

Harriet and Nokomis. Following the banks of the Mississippi River before crossing into Saint Paul, miles 21-25 proceed on a steady uphill from the river where the race finishes at the Minnesota State Capitol. Tree-lined throughout, with the fall colors above your head and under your feet, it is a small-town-feel race with thousands and thousands of spectators.

No matter what your day is like, the downhill last half-mile allows for a strong finish which can often make the whole effort feel worth it.

My Experience:

After a month of two marathons in Europe, a half marathon in Utah, a triathlon in Oregon and a business trip to Vegas, I would hardly say I was in good shape to run this race. Well-meaning friends who just "know" you are going to do "good" are just that: well-meaning. You thank them and know that you are a wiped-out and tired mess. But going into this marathon the promises of 40-50-degree weather with cloudy skies meant that I would be running in the best weather for a race in... let me see... oh yeah... forever.

As a guest of the race, I was able to spend some time with some elites at the hotel before it started. I was not the slowest person there but I am fairly certain any whom I may have been faster than had at least two decades on me. I walked to the start with Michael Wardian, one of the best runners out there at being able to take on short distances, marathons, and ultras, all week after week. His stamina and versatility are quite amazing. I also met a new friend named Mike who, I didn't know at the time, was dealing with some pretty bad foot issues. We chatted away and just tried to enjoy the fact that the race was slightly chilly and the atmosphere was fantastic. Then we parted ways as they did last minute strides and prepped for running blazingly fast. I went to the bathroom and stood around looking at people. Oh, the dichotomy.

I was close to the front of the race due to my "elite" bib and I knew

Race: Twin Cities Marathon

Typical Date: First Weekend in October

Distance: Marathon

Location: Minneapolis / Saint Paul

Why You Should Run It:

When I think about recommending a race to others I ask them about two different things: are they looking to run a good time or are they looking to have a good time? Very few races offer both except for the fact that running a good time can often trump whether you had a good time along the course. Having said that, the Twin Cities Marathon is not an easy course. It is not exceedingly difficult either, especially in today's world of making races difficult for difficulty's sake. However, if you wish to be involved in a race which is very well-run, extremely well-supported, and showcases two beautiful urban areas in the United States, you would be hard pressed to find anything much better than this race. Will you run a good time? Perhaps, but you will work for it. Will you have a good time? The odds are highly likely you will.

Originally called the Land of Lakes Marathon when it was founded in 1975, five participants, all male, raced the 26.2-mile trek along Minneapolis' streets and parkways. It was renamed the City of Lakes Marathon and moved to a four-lap course around Lake Calhoun and Lake Harriet. In 1981, the race had grown but Saint Paul also had its own marathon as well. The next year, realizing a marathon which connected Minneapolis to Saint Paul and combined the spectacular autumn beauty of both cities would be greater attraction than two competing marathons on either side of the Mississippi River, the inaugural Twin Cities Marathon was established.

The course runs through downtown Minneapolis for the first portions of the race including around Lake of the Isles, Calhoun, many would either be running faster than me or going out too fast. As such, I was unsurprised when dozens upon dozens streamed past me in the first few miles. I did my best to hold myself in check and simply tried to go out at a sub-three-hour pace. The first mile was a little hot so I gladly backed off the throttle. A surprising hill at mile two helped me do just that and suddenly I was right where I needed to be.

The sheer number of people around me was startling. I did the math and found out that you would have to combine the last 16 marathons I have run to get more finishers (9,727) than would finish the Twin Cities Marathon alone (8,579). I had, for the most part, been running essentially training runs with no one around me for three years and getting a finisher's medal when I did it. That is a hard way to race. Having runners pushing me was a blessing. Having so many others around me was a bit of a nuisance.

As we hit the third mile and began to skirt the Lake of the Isles, two things would soon become evident. The first was the first half of this marathon consisted of many small bends in the road which made running the tangents essential to not running well over 26.2 miles. Having so many others around you makes this rather tiring. You have to spend a great deal of mental energy trying to pick a path through the runners. At least you have to if you don't want to be a jerk, that is, and don't just plow through others. No matter how fast I am running, my speed will always take a seat when it comes to race etiquette.

The second thing which was clear was no matter what I tried, no matter how much I surged or laid off the throttle, I was going to run right around seven-minute miles. Without fail, every mile passed by and I expected something either much faster or much slower based on the effort it took to run that mile. However, time and time again, seven minutes per mile popped up on my watch. As I knew seven minutes per mile equaled a 3:03:33 (one of those random things I remember about marathon pace) I figured that I might as well stick with this as long as I could. If a sub-three wasn't in the cards, there is no sense trying for it and bonking. I didn't want to run a 3:33:33.

Run This Place

Passing by Lake Calhoun, we were onto a slimmer road where the jostling of runners became a little dicier. However, despite being wary of the extra runners, I was enjoying myself. In fact, each mile that went by at almost exactly seven minutes started to tickle me. I began to think of a race I ran where no matter what I tried, I ran almost the exact same pace mile after mile. Trying to recall exactly which helped passed the time.[133] The thing about the marathon is that even at a good clip, you have three hours to be alone with your thoughts. If you run it correctly, you are more or less spending two hours of controlled running until you get to the nitty gritty where you push. So often you are just biding time until those two hours are gone. With me, I like to think about stats.

After passing Lake Harriet there was a funny yet cruel spectator sign which said we were 28% done. The fact we weren't yet even a third done was overshadowed by the randomness of "28%." Around here I began to hear the chatter of a group behind me. As I would come to learn, this was the 3:05 pace group. Why they were so close to me here confused me. Perhaps the desired pace was to run even effort and they would slow on the hills near the end of the race. Banking time, so to speak, is a strategy which almost never works. For some reason I started to worry for these runners, relying on a pacer who may be taking them out too fast. In addition, I wasn't fond of a herd of runners right on my heels. So, I picked up the pace, turned on the afterburners… and ran the exact same mile again.

We spent the next few miles on the Minnehaha Parkway next to the Minnehaha Creek.[134] Even here, in a relatively out of the way place, the amazing spectators were lining the course. As sick of cowbells as I am (especially when they are wrung *at* you) the energy and fervor of the people lived up to its reputation. I can unequivocally state that throughout the course, my spirits were exponentially raised by those urging the runners onward. As I mentioned above, it had been a long time since I felt this lift. It did not go unappreciated.

---

[133] I only had 82 half marathons and 155 marathons to go over in my mind.
[134] I was just Minnehahappy to be there.

After the tenth mile, the 3:05 pace group passed me. I was astonished. I decided to hang with them for the remainder of the mile to experiment. I wanted to see if I could keep up their pace and exactly what pace they were running. When we hit mile eleven and I ran a 6:57 (a 3:02 marathon pace) I just shook my head. Whatever the plan of this pace group was, I didn't understand it and wasn't going to hang around. I slowed down and expected to fall back into my previous tempo.

But suddenly it was as if the group, which just began to disappear in front of me, had stuck a needle in my body and sucked out all the energy I had. My next two miles to the half, both way slower than I expected, left me dumbfounded. I tried not to think about this and instead focused my energy elsewhere. We circumvented Lake Nokomis and I looked at the waters wistfully. I wondered if it would have been more fun to be in a canoe on one of the lakes today than out here running.

I have often said that mile fourteen is one of the most important miles in a marathon. After the boost of passing through the halfway point, this mile can often set the tone for the rest of the race. There is always the chance for a letdown after the half marathon point and if you run a strong fourteenth mile, then you can hopefully ride that to the end. Then I ran 23 seconds slower than I wanted to run. Ooof.

Fortunately, the fifteenth mile was much better and I hoped that I had just experienced a weird three-mile lull. Running alongside the Mississippi River would be wonderful if you could in fact tell you were running alongside the Mississippi River. I often hear people tell tales of their races and they sound like travel agencies. They mention how it is near this body of water or this mountain or what have you. But in reality, while it is technically very close to those things, you often can't actually see the sights. All it takes is a line of trees or a slight mound of dirt to obstruct the view of virtually anything. I was hoping for something to feast my eyes upon to perhaps pick up my spirits but saw none. Then as my next few miles continued to slow, I no longer even tried to observe the beautiful homes to our left or the mighty Mississippi to our right. Instead, my mind was whirling as I attempted to decipher what time I would run if I kept up the present pace. Math always distracts but it often does not give you the answer you are hoping for in a marathon.

Throughout the race there were a series of small hills. Nothing substantial but a plethora of them and while they may be small they were mighty.[135] At the eighteenth mile, I walked up one of them for a bit. These ten seconds of walking slowed my pace but seemed to waken my legs. The next two miles, while crossing the river and then heading to the last 10K, were the fastest in half an hour. Perhaps I could keep up the pace and garner a respectable 3:06 marathon time.

Unfortunately, I did not know what hills remained.

If you look at the elevation profile of the course, it hardly looks that daunting. Most of those hills I mentioned in the first half are almost imperceptible. And from mile 21-23, the hill which undoubtedly crushed the hopes and dreams of many is barely a 150-footer. But woe unto those who do not take these hills seriously. The Summit Street that runners are on from mile 22 to virtually the end is aptly named. Even though I ran two miles far slower than I would like I began to pass runner after runner.

While the weather was cool, the sun was shining brightly. Without a doubt this ELSO[136] would have worn heavily on runners if not for how wonderfully shaded we were on this course. I would say 85% of the race provided cover of some sort. Here on Summit Street it was no different. A wetter-than-normal summer kept the trees from being their usually vibrant and beautiful colors, but the leaves were appreciated to no end.

Finally cresting the hill with a 5K left I was ready for what had been promised to me by spectators — an all downhill finish. Spectators lie. More rolling hills continued to pop up here and there every time I thought we were done with the climbs. I did the math and

---

[135] Thank you, Bard.
[136] Evil Life Sucking Orb.

realized that I was not going to get any particular time I was hoping to get. In fact, if I didn't hunker down I would not be getting a Boston Qualifying time. I was not going to let that happen.

It has been quite some time since I have been able to really ignore pain, fatigue and suffering, and slip into pain vision. This is what I call the narrowing of the eyes and the focusing on virtually nothing but a white line on the pavement in front of me. While my pace did not exactly quicken, I was passing dozens of runners.[137] That said, I cared not one bit about what place I finished or who I passed. I wanted a time that was under 3:10.

Hitting mile 26 under a huge American flag showed me I had about ten seconds to spare at my current pace. Not wishing to risk it if the mile marker was a touch off, I picked up the pace. My eyes were on the clock and I saw its red blinking evil eye tick upward unmercifully. Finally, with a few meters to go I knew my hard work in the last few miles would pay off. I crossed under the finish line in 3:09:49 for my 55th fastest marathon ever. It was also my 16th 3:09 marathon.[138]

A crisp cool day surrounded by lakes and trees with completely random strangers whom you will never see again in your life,[139] screaming their heads off for you for the five seconds they see you. Hometown-feel with big city know-how. That's the Twin Cities Marathon.

Running is not the cure for all that ails you. In addition, America is not a perfect place. But while running this marathon in cities which are so different it is hard to understand why they are called twins on a beautiful fall day makes you think maybe this sport is as close to perfect as we are going to get, even if just for a few hours on a Sunday in October.

---

[137] 82 in the last five miles according to the stats provided post-race.
[138] That's what you get when you pace the 3:10 group so many times.
[139] And Candice, who found me to tell me she had beat me by about a minute.

Race: Fargo Marathon

Typical Date: Fourth Sunday in June

Distance: Half marathon

Location: Fargo, ND

Why You Should Run It:

Putting on a marathon is an exhausting, and often thankless, task. That is when everything goes right. So when in late March 2010 precipitation in various forms flooded the Red River in Fargo to record heights, doubts about whether the Fargo Marathon would be even run immediately cropped up. Volunteers, townspeople and paid workers toiled endlessly to shore up dikes and make new walls to hold back the surging water. They weren't doing this to save the marathon but rather to save their homes and the town.

Having said that, their efforts were indicative of what the marathon committee itself was doing to save a race about to enter its fifth year. With Herculean planning at the eleventh hour, the Fargo Marathon assured all its runners the race would go on, albeit slightly modified in nature. Instead of heading over to Moorhead, Minnesota across the surging Red River, the race would now stay completely in Fargo, making two laps of the same 13.1 course.

I tell you this because the Fargo Marathon you run will be different. Your fans won't be able to stand in one place and see you something akin to eight different times. But this type of energy, to put together a race for their runners when no sensible person would have faulted them for saying "Not this year, sorry!" is admirable and indicative of one of those intangibles that makes a race must-run.

Often I lament how a race which runs through neighborhoods is often bereft of, well, neighbors. But Fargo takes this race seriously and thousands of residents come out to cheer runners on. With a race course starting and ending inside the FargoDome[140], running along the Red River, trek through three college campuses, and being flat without being too flat, you can see why this is one of my favorites.

My Experience:

This marathon was my fifth marathon in four weeks in the middle of my greatest stretch of marathon running to date. I was asked to be the 3:10 pace group leader and have always loved being able to do that for fellow runners. At the time it was the fastest qualifying time for Boston and I took great pride in helping others reach their goal.

I told the runners assembled around me it is nearly impossible to take the first mile slow. Crowd excitement, revved engines, and goals in the mind push you forward too fast far too often. So when we hit the first mile dead on, I was stoked. Then we went eleven seconds too fast on the second mile. Whoops. But the next few miles were exact and I could feel the group collectively relax as they finally believed they were in good hands.

When we hit the 10K, I whipped a cellphone out of my pocket and called my buddy GP Pearlberg who was announcing at the finish line. I wanted him to know the 3:10 group was right on pace.[141] Someone asked if I was calling my wife and I said: "My bald British male friend will get a kick out of that one!" GP put his phone up to the mic and apparently the crowd enjoyed the reply.

With my pack firmly in charge of the roads, we began to really settle into pace. Almost every mile was what we needed which was hard to do for a number of reasons. First, the course was so flat and easy that my runners were champing at the bit. Often I would get swallowed up by the pack as runners would push by me in their eagerness to finish. Then like clockwork I would watch them look back over their shoulder in slight panic to see me

---

[140] Weather in Fargo in May ranges as greatly as just about any other so having bathrooms indoors and a finish there as well is something which should not be undersold.
[141] Yes, I will admit this was nothing short of hubris and silliness on my part.

behind them and fall back again. As we could continually hit each mile right on the desired pace, I would sort of give them a smug look like "See?"

Second, the crowds were fantastic. For those who had only run in big city races or were running one of their first marathons, they had no idea how spectacular the crowds were. People lined almost every square inch of the 13.1-mile loop. Part of this had to do with the fact that because of the two-loop nature of the course fans knew they would see not only the half marathon runners but the marathoners twice in the exact same spot (and sometimes double that as we ran up and then back down a street a few miles later). The other fact had to do with the civic pride that Fargo had in its marathon. I spoke to a volunteer afterward who told me a usual conversation around town that weekend was whether you were going to run the marathon, help put on the marathon, or cheer for the marathon. There seemed to be no other option for the townspeople. With a population of only around 90,000, I bet two out of every nine people in the city were lining the streets.

As we neared the FargoDome to begin our second loop, I told those in my group that we now knew what lay ahead. No surprises and no reason to worry. I expected that my pack of twenty-strong would be whittled in half when the half marathoners took their turn to finish in the warm and friendly confines of the FargoDome. Imagine my surprise when nearly every runner in my pack stayed with me as we began our second loop.

I started telling my runners some of my trade secrets for staying focused through these next miles.[142] It is the second half of a marathon where my inner mother goose comes out and I take the finishing of all "my runners" personally. Yet they cared about me, too. At one point, a runner behind me noticed I had a splotch of blood on my sock and had apparently been watching it grow for a few miles. I told him I could feel some chafing but had no choice to run on. His reply was "Nice sock, Schilling!"[143]

---

[142] I hope no one ate bad Indian food last night.
[143] For those not getting the reference, my sports-minded runner was alluding to the blood seeping from Curt Schilling's sock in the 2004 baseball playoffs

As the miles passed by my group stayed tight. When the wind would whip up they would heed my advice and use me as a shield. We lost a runner here and there as one fell back or surged ahead but a solid group of about seven or eight stuck together as the miles ticked by. Each mile brought us closer to our goal; a shared goal even though it meant so many different things to so many people.

With about a mile left, as always happens, those with the desire to get this darn race over with, pushed ahead. Their goal was not to hit 3:10 right on the nose but rather break 3:10 or get as close as possible and not pass out at the end. The finish line and that specific time was often what they had been dreaming about for months and working hard for mile after mile on this day.

As they left me, for about half a mile I was alone. I then came upon this sprite-like female who I had seen pass us miles before. I could tell she was struggling and a post-race analysis of her times proved this (she slowed considerable in the last 10K). With no one else around me to pace I slowed my step a bit and began to encourage her to continue the best I could. She picked up the pace for few hundred yards but then quickly fell back. I repeated my cheering, she sped up, and then slowed down. Pick up, back off. I could tell that she was obviously going to qualify for Boston but I also knew she was hoping to break into the 3:10s. However, up ahead I saw another runner who had been right by my side for miles and miles. For about ten steps I saw his pace slack and now I knew I had a new charge to get to finish line.

As we neared mile 26, I had slowed by a good 15 seconds off the previous pace in an effort to help that female runner. Bill was this runner's name and I could see he wanted that BQ more than anything else in the world. My showing up by his side lit a fire under him and away he went. He left me in the dust over the next quarter of a mile and I smiled. Two more runners who had been with me earlier, Scott and Brandon, appeared at my side, and I

---

where he famously pitched just hours after having surgery on his ankle and receiving a cadaver's tendon in the process. Schilling has since become a right-wing conspiracy theory nutjob. But in 2010 he was still ok.

now had two more reasons to run hard.

Around the outside of FargoDome, down the ramp and into the final 100 yards we ran. I thought I might have a chance of an exact 3:10 but at the time I did not care. With fans cheering from the stands and a carnival-like atmosphere all around us, every runner felt like a rock star.

We sprinted across the finish and began high-fiving and hugging. I found Bill who was beside himself with glee and he just thanked me over and over again. I handed him the 3:10 sign which I had been holding for hours and told him he deserved it. You would have thought I had given him a Ferrari.

Dane Rauschenberg

Race: Whidbey Island Marathon

Typical Date: Mid-April

Distance: Marathon

Location: Whidbey Island, WA

Why You Should Run It:

Just north of Seattle, nestled up in Washington State's Puget Sound, is Whidbey Island. Starting at the famed Deception Pass Bridge[144] then winding its way through picturesque ocean views and tranquil farmland, the course switches from country back-roads to waterfront coastlines, with snow-capped mountains in the background and a series of challenging hills under your feet. It is entirely possible to see orcas, eagles, seals, and deer on this course. Good luck finding those four on any other 26.2 miles of running.

I am going to make special note of those challenging hills because often when people think of running on an island, hills don't come to mind. They are quite present on Whidbey and you best familiarize yourself with them. The inclines at miles nine and seventeen are particularly grueling, with portions of the latter at a seven percent grade. The course reaches its highest point at the eighteen-mile mark, after which it's downhill to mile twenty-three and flat to the finish at Windjammer Park. But with mid-April weather in the great Seattle area almost always being darn near perfect for a marathon, even a few long hills are bearable.

My Experience:

The morning broke absolutely gorgeously. If I was doing anything else besides running a marathon, I would have been in heaven. Bright sunshine, regardless of the temperature, is not my ideal

[144] So called because Captain George Vancouver, when exploring the area in the 1790s, didn't realize Whidbey was an island, not a peninsula. Maybe it should be called "Wait Until You Know What Something Is Before Naming It Bridge".

race condition. Fortunately, as I would learn through the course, there was a great deal of shade provided by trees, hills, and houses along the way. As such, only a few sections were totally exposed to the elements. Given that not one single cloud darted across the sky on this day that was a good thing.

An appreciated amenity provided by the race was shuttles from the hotels to the race start and from the end of the race to the hotels. Very little planning was needed transportation-wise, which is excellent for a point-to-point race. As the race started, we went down the slightest of hills before beginning the first of many rises, this one leading to aforementioned Deception Pass Bridge. Describing how beautiful this morning and this bridge were exceeds my capabilities.[145] My head was on a swivel as I looked at both sides of the bridge, the water below, the eddying tides, the rocks which were hewn out by the passage of time and everything else I could take in. The bridge was far too short for my liking.

At this juncture I was about in fifteenth place and felt like I wasn't pressing. When I ran this race I was in the middle of the worst year of racing I have ever experienced. With a left calf muscle barely functioning, it wasn't the wisest idea to have even started this marathon. Sometimes we do unwise things.

Around the third or fourth mile I slipped into this odd Nyquil-like-induced fog. A strange fuzziness took over. Given I had never really felt anything of the sort before it was both intriguing and a tad worrisome. Eventually, it subsided and as perplexing as it was, I never found an answer to its cause.

A few runners passed me near the 10K mark and I passed a few who had been in front of me. One of the female leaders had already stopped to tie her shoe and stretch out a calf muscle. I felt bad for her to be dealing with this so early in the race. But no sooner did I emote about her situation then she sprung up and disappeared into the distance. So much for sympathy for the speedy!

---

[145] That's probably a bad thing since I am a writer.

Having barely run anything over thirteen miles in the previous few months I was happy with how I was feeling in this opening portion. I was also cautiously aware that this might get ugly. As we traversed a long wonderful downhill, skirting a slew of waterfront houses for sale on Skagit Bay that were priced to move, the first sign of my leg giving me some trouble showed up.[146] Nevertheless, the views were breathtaking. The mountains of both Olympic National Park and Mt Baker in the Snoqualmie National Forest were off in the distance on two different sides. On this crystal clear day one could see for hundreds of miles from this vantage point. It really was astounding. My running, on the other hand, was not.

As the course flattened, I found this was the only time I could actually speed up at all. Normally I can cruise the downhill portions, laying waste to anyone who was able to pass me on the up. Here, however, a pain began to grow in my groin and quad. I realized that extending or accelerating on hills was not going to happen. Given the amount of hills on this course, this wasn't ideal.

The flat section before the monster hill at the ninth mile only made the climb that much more wearisome. What I thought would be a problem on that day, a lack of energy in later miles from undertraining, never became an issue. Perhaps it was the forced slower pace but throughout the day, energy was aplenty. The climb right at mile ten got so ridiculously steep I heard someone drop, under their breath, a "mother farmer." I actually laughed out loud as I thought the same thing when I saw it.[147]

A little kick for me personally was when Ryan, a pre-teen who I had met at the race expo the day before and who was an unbelievably

---

[146] As a sidebar "Skagit" has to be one of the most awful names for anything ever. Later when I saw there was a Skagit Public Utility District called the Skagit PUD I realized I think I found the worst name of a place to ever work in history. Even when I learned that "Skagit" is pronounced with a soft "g" it only made it minorly less offensive to the ear.

[147] It went up ~95 feet in a tenth of a mile. I thought they were going to give us Sherpas and a rope guide to help get us up and over.

fast runner in his own right, left me a sign on the side of the road to inspire me as a surprise. The hill was still just as tough but at least I smiled a little.

Once over the hill, I finally felt robust in my running. Under our feet was a much more reasonable downhill portion, allowing me to pick up my pace. I would be remiss if I did not mention I had already taken three bathroom breaks in the first 10K. I was happy I hadn't needed to take another until mile 12 because they were getting a little ridiculous. I've been asked if I had ever been nauseated or had to use the bathroom during a race and, if so, why I thought that was. I've always replied I have gone through every physical ailment one could possibly imagine. For the most part, wondering why something is happening is futile. Just deal with it when it happens and try to learn from it.[148]

I knew the next seven miles would challenge me. At mile twelve we saw the mile twenty marker on the other side of the road so we knew we would be coming back down this way. But as good as I had felt at miles thirteen and fourteen, miles fifteen and sixteen almost did me in. A very long downhill only served as a reminder that my leg was not working properly.

Yet, like before, in spite of the pain in my groin, I had no problem climbing the hills. Many who would go on to beat me soundly were forced to walk a few of these. The pain in my leg had gone away but the "not wanting to be out here anymores" were kicking in. As a few more runners passed me, runners I know should not have been doing so, I just had to suck it in, enjoy the beautiful day, and use my extra energy to cheer on all the other runners on the other side of the road about to take on the massive hills in front of them.

I distinctly recall looking at my watch at mile 21 and seeing that at that point it was only 12 seconds faster than my marathon PR. Knowing I still had five miles left when normally I would be done

---

[148] So, in other words, if you have to pee every 15 minutes for the first hour of a race, then go and pee.

was a bit of a kick to the huevos. Looming ahead of us was another mountain of a hill which I did not recall being on the course map. Fortunately, we turned right before it and I breathed a huge sigh of relief. I knew the hill at mile 24 was all I could handle.

A slight jaunt through what I am guessing was military housing had more than a few people out cheering us on. There was also at least one unplanned aid station from a little brother and sister team who were handing out full bottles of water. That was just awesome.

A flat section on a very wide bicycle path which ran flush with the bay was absolutely beautiful. Too bad I was now in such pain I couldn't fully enjoy it. I began to wonder if I had done permanent damage. After talking about how to 'Do Nothing Foolish' to so many people, I wondered if I had. Then the final cruel hill popped up in front of me. Again, many were slowed to a crawl. Suddenly, my groin felt better; I took the hill with gusto and began passing people who had passed me. Before I knew it I was up and over and heading to the last mile.

As I traversed this last mile, I could hear the footsteps of another runner behind me. They were letting me cut a swatch through the runners, complete with my "On your left!"s and their over-exaggerated jumps and surprised yells to make me feel like the bad guy. I was tempted to let my trailing runner pass me as I knew I wasn't really in the best shape for a sprint to the finish.

For the entire last mile, whenever I could hear or feel them surge, I would do the same. Only in the finish chute when the half marathoners blatantly did not follow the "marathoners to the right; halfs to the left" signs and I had to stutter step to get around a large group, did I finally succumb. The runner passed me and took me by about one second at the finish line. I finished 42nd overall in a time of 3:34:19 which was my 137th slowest of 148 lifetime marathons. If one can be satisfied with a result and disappointed at the same time, this was that.

But I licked my wounds, saw they were not permanent, and then immediately was awash in the natural beauty around me. Having conquered this demon of a course with non-functioning legs felt amazing.

Race: Marine Corps Marathon

Typical Date: Last Sunday in October

Distance: Marathon

Location: Arlington, VA and Washington, D.C.

Why You Should Run It:

Oprah.

I'm kidding. But chances are you know this race because of Ms. Winfrey, even if you don't know that is why you do. Her 1994 finish of the Marine Corps Marathon more or less jumpstarted the second boom of running. This boom included all of the people who previously wouldn't even dream of running a marathon if they couldn't break four hours. Now, the most egalitarian of sports, running embraces all, no matter how slow.[149]

So yeah, Oprah is part of it. So are the actual Marines. The ones who run many of the aid stations, provide course security, and, most importantly, put the medal around your neck when you are finished. Marines are the everyman who become the best of what many of us hope to be. Fittingly, the Marine Corps Marathon is known as the People's Marathon because it continues to embrace that same everyman mantra. There is no prize money. No big-name runners show up. It is not an exceptionally fast course.[150] Just a week before the much-more ballyhooed New York City Marathon with its "Um, we're New York" type attitude, this far less-presumptuous, yet still sixth-largest marathon in the U.S., takes a back seat to no one when it comes to making everyone feel like a star.

---

[149] Some would argue, with good reason, that perhaps the marathon is not for everyone and putting such an emphasis on it, and just completing it has made the accomplishment a little less special. Discuss.

[150] It is also constantly changing because of safety factors, construction, growing number of participants, etc.

Run This Place

Even if you live in the greater D.C. area and run there all the time, there is something about trotting past some of our most precious historical monuments, unfettered by normally snarling traffic, which cannot be beat. The statues look taller, brighter, and cleaner on race day than any other day. Then when you finish up a hill to the Marine Corps War Memorial and get to have one who helps keep this country safe put a medal around your neck, well, you would be hard-pressed to have bigger butterflies in your stomach.

My Experience:

The Marine Corps Marathon is the only marathon that I have run five separate times. My first experience with this race was when I ran it as my third marathon ever. It was also the third consecutive time I had bonked severely in a marathon and seriously considered never running another again. Yet, inexplicably I had signed up for another 26.2-mile race just three weeks later in nearby Maryland. That race, run in extremely cold weather, showed me what I needed was just some lower temperatures to do well. As such, for the next three years in which I lived in Arlington, Virginia, where the second mile of this race was one block from my home, I made the Marine Corps Marathon my yearly pilgrimage.

In fact, this race almost holds the distinction of being the second race where I ran faster every time I competed in it.[151] Given how poorly I ran the first rendtion it is not surprising that I improved the second time I ran it. But I did not just improve; I set a new personal best of 3:07:25 which bested a PR from earlier in the year. That race was my final marathon before I ran 52 in a row the next year. Yes, I went from thinking I would never run another marathon again to four months later being knee-deep in the preparation for a year's worth of weekly 26.2-milers.

When I ran it as part of my 52 in a row, I did not set a personal best. However, I did run my second fastest time ever. The only faster race was my first ever sub-three-hour marathon the

---

[151] The first being the Blossom Time Run profiled earlier in this book. The Carlsbad Marathon falls short on a technicality as I ran the 3:10 pace group there for three years and ran a 3:09:50; 3:09:52 and 3:09:52. Yeah, this guy paces.

weekend prior at the Niagara Falls Marathon. Here, in my 43rd marathon of the year, I ran a 3:03:54. The next year, my last as a greater D.C. resident, I ran a 2:55:34 and set a new personal best.

I took a three-year break from the race after and did not run it again until 2010. That year, I hadn't been back to D.C. in a few years and forgot about how difficult it can be to get to the starting line. Normally, I just ran down the hill. This time, however, I was staying with some friends in Alexandria and tried to make use of the Metro. As it was a mildly chilly morning, I wore a shirt I didn't want to throw away, along with my car keys and other accoutrements. I utilized the bag drop for the first time, or tried to at least. Unfortunately, I got off at the wrong stop and left myself not nearly enough time to get to the appropriate place to drop my bag. In fact, when the giant Howitzer gun fired to signify the start of the marathon I was still half a mile away from the drop-off. Dashing madly to the trucks, I heaved my bag into the back of one of them before scrambling back to the start. While the race was a chip-timed event, the last thing I wanted to do was have to pick my way through roughly 20,000 runners.

By the time I got to the timing mat, I had run an extra 1.5 miles. I tried to settle into my race but it was hard shaking the feeling that I had already expended too much energy. After a few miles, I knew my pre-race goal of another PR was out the window. Nevertheless, I was still having a fairly decent race, once I calmed down. I slowed a touch after the first half but with my knowledge of the course, I felt I could make a charge for a fast finish.

Fast forward to mile twenty-three, when I passed through Crystal City and could see runners heading back our way on the other side of the street. I thought how happy I would be if I was just about a minute ahead of where I was presently, running alongside them. I had been using one particular female runner in front of me as measure of my pace. We had both been picking off runners on a warm but not too hot day. Then it happened.

As I approached the 24th mile, every ounce of energy left my

Run This Place

body. I don't even call it "hitting the wall." I call it falling through a trap door. Suddenly, ferociously, and without any real warning, my race was done. I walked through an aid station drinking thoroughly from the cups provided; fully hoping it would sustain me for roughly fifteen more minutes of running. I knew I had lost some time but if I hit mile 24 in a 7:45 mile, maybe I could power though, use my endurance, and run two sub-seven-minute miles to get a 3:02.[152] When I passed mile 24 my watch told me my fate: 8:18 for this mile. NOW, the race was done.

I began to shuffle and walk and jog and curse. Around the lonely Pentagon parking lot, up an off ramp, and down another lonely stretch before coming down an off ramp on the other side of the Pentagon, I trotted. I was pretty peeved, to be honest. I knew that right around mile 26 of running, if you count my pre-race jog, my body had stopped. It was like "Hey, we have done our job. What more do you want?"

I passed the 25th mile and just wanted it to be over. I could see the long stretch of highway in front of me and passed the spot where I had dropped my bag about three hours prior. Time slipped away and my 7:00 miles became 9:30 minute miles. Oh well. One last hill. No victory celebration for me today. The only saving grace was to run another 3:09 and qualify for Boston again. I am not pooh-poohing that achievement but it definitely was not what I was shooting for. Marines lined the finishing chute and I could see them ahead handing out medals. I crossed the finish line and almost instantly stopped. Actually, I think I stopped about a foot in front of the finish and my momentum carried me forward.

In either case, any marathon finished upright and official is a celebration. That's something one can say later. At the time most thoughts contain swear words.

---

[152] Why 3:02? As I mentioned earlier, I was playing the "knock out a specific time" game. When I ran this race in 2010, I had never run a 3:02 and that was the only time above three hours I hadn't been able to snag. Yes, I am a dork.

Race: Quad Cities Marathon

Typical Date: Last Sunday in September

Distance: Marathon

Location: Davenport, IA

Why You Should Run It:

The course is not particularly beautiful, although it has its moments. The crowds aren't ten deep but they have their spots. The weather is a little volatile but can be fine. But the organizers put on one of the best races in America and for those who are stuck on bling or mountain visages and do not realize what really makes a race tick are all the things you haven't the foggiest clue go on behind the scenes, you should go with the people that make those things work. That is the Quad Cities Marathon for you.

Four cities, three bridges, two states, and one island, all along the mighty Mississippi River.

Posting an APB for a Diet Mountain Dew and having not one but two separate people from the Quad Cities bringing me one at my booth just goes to show you what sort of awesome people live here. (Also, seriously, Mountain Dew, I do more for you than X Games. Hook a brother up.)

My Experience:

I have run this race four times: twice the marathon and twice the half. I was supposed to make it a fifth but a random aggravated assault a few weeks before the race left me with a fractured face and three pins in my thumb.[153] But the experience which sticks me the most is when I ran the Quad Cities Marathon the day after finishing a 165-mile run from Dane, Wisconsin to Davenport, IA.

---

[153] Cut to my Dad: "Do you run with your face or thumb?" N.B. My father passed in 2012 and never said this but it is the type of thing he would say to get me to chuckle.

I had always wanted to visit Dane, the only city in America which shares my name, but never had a real reason to do so. So, I concocted a three-day run starting in Dane, stopping to talk to kids at schools and people various functions along the way about chasing their dreams, before ending in Davenport, Iowa. I would take on the role as the speaker at the pre-race dinner and run a marathon the next day. It would be a heck of a test.

I can count on one hand the number of times in 145 marathons run heading into this day where I was even remotely close to not wanting to run as I was when I woke up the morning of this race. I was exhausted. I was sick. I did not want to leave the bed. Whether it was illness brought on from being tired or exhaustion brought on from being sick, I know it took everything I had to get out of the hotel. A little bit of dry-heaving seconds before I left definitely did little to persuade me. It also surprised the heck out of me. All I had was my usual strawberry milk and my body was rejecting it.

Somehow I got going and found myself walking to the start with my expansive and numerous crew for the Dane to Davenport.[154] She was also running the marathon after safely helping me navigate my run and I can only imagine how tired she was. After making sure I got to the finish line of my three-day trek, with just as little sleep as I had, all while tending to all my needs, I knew she wasn't at her best either. But in spite of a bad foot, a week's worth of travel, and ushering me around the expo for both a book signing and a speech the night before the race, she was heading out the door.

We parted ways at the corrals and I tried to steady myself for the upcoming 26.2. Could I do it in roughly a Boston Qualifying time? Would it take me north of four hours to traverse the course? Or would I be somewhere in between? I really and truly had no idea what to expect.

Running a pace much slower than normal for me, I was experiencing a totally different race. I have often talked about how two runners in the same race on the same day can have two

---

[154] One person, my good friend, Shannon.

completely separate experiences. While the Porta-Potties were plentiful, I was always getting to them right as another person was entering one or I could see they were already occupied. They were normally free for me to use, unhindered by these awful people who dared to think they too could enjoy race amenities.

Suddenly, I felt fantastic. I began passing runners and picking up the pace. The next three miles felt wonderful and thought perhaps it only took me a bit of warming up to get my engine running. I passed a guy wearing violent green toe-shoes and thought "Well, at least that guy isn't going to beat me." Going up over the bridge slowed me a bunch and Ninja Turtle Toe Shoe guy slid by. It is hard to dislike a person because of their shoe choice but it is hard to run 165 miles in three days and I did that.[155] Luckily, the downside of the bridge into Rock Island allowed me to repass him. Now, I didn't hate him so much.

But just as suddenly as I felt great, I felt bad again. The next mile or so had me really beginning to wonder if I could even finish. I debated a small walking break to gather myself. The weight of the previous 165 miles really was taking its toll. I wasn't all that sore. I was just wrung.the.heck.out. And then Toe Shoes passed me again.

Around the 12th mile I tried to pick it up and was rewarded with a stop, grab your knees and vomit situation. Twice I dry heaved a whole lot of nothing but pride. I wondered if I might have my first marathon DNF ever. My situation was getting atrocious. But I pulled myself together and gathered my wits. I relied on good ole math tricks to distract me. I knew the last six miles were an out-and-back along the very same road I had finished the Dane to Davenport. All I needed to do was get to mile 20. That was only seven miles. I could walk these final thirteen if necessary.

Another bridge took us onto the Rock Island Arsenal and I was halfway done. Hang on, big fella. Only one more bridge to go. Not soon after entering the Arsenal, we joined half marathoners coming from a different direction. More math games were played

[155] So what I am saying is don't doubt my abilities to do the absurd.

and more miles passed by. I needed to use the bathroom again. When I finally spotted a Porta-Potty, I saw another runner slip inside of it. I saw I had about thirty seconds of running to get there and hoped he would be done by the time I arrived. He wasn't. I waited. I made loud throat-clearing noises. Finally, I just had to leave. I couldn't wait any longer.

Once again we joined the half marathoners, who hadn't done the same tour of the Arsenal which we had. Once again I had to skirt a fine line between running over the five-abreasters and running in the other lane of traffic. Luckily, the other lane was on this military installation and there wasn't another car coming our way. Nevertheless, I was doing my best not to break laws around people who are allowed to carry firearms.

I readied myself for the final bridge crossing and onto mile 20, and was met with a sobering visage. Up ahead, two police cars were pulled to the side and the officers were administering feverish chest compressions to a downed runner. It was an awful sight to see. I could see the body language of every runner who wanted to do something, anything, but did not know what to do. I finally decided to let the men in blue do their thing and keep going. Fortunately, it appears this runner, Jeff B, was saved by these fine officers and will live to run another day. I did not know this cheery outcome at the time and I can say it was a bitter pill to swallow. Who cares about running this far when I might have just watched a person die? But, I had no choice but to press forward.

By now, some of the elites were heading back to the finish. I did some math and realized that when I hit mile 21, if I had been running my marathon personal best, I would have been done. That crushed the spirit a bit. But what lifted it was seeing many runners who had passed me earlier, or who had been in front of me for miles, coming back into focus. I pushed forward with an eye towards doing nothing rash or stupid.

Unfortunately, my math brain kicked in and I realized I had an off chance to get a sub 3:30. You see, at this point, I had completed 145 marathons and 130 of them have been under 3:30. I pride myself on not simply completing marathons but giving all I have at the time. Granted this was indeed all I had but to get anything within a "3:2x" time would just be the icing on the cake. I promised myself that the last four miles would be consecutively faster.

It ended up that not only the last four miles but the last six were consecutively faster. Also, at mile 25 I passed Mr. Toe Shoes. I would be a liar if I said that did not feel particularly good. With just about .2 to go, Joe Moreno, the race director for Quad Cities and a guy you wish you could clone to either run or help direct every race out there, appeared by my side. I decided I wanted to pick it up and see if he could sprint next to me. He started laughing and kept pace, so I picked it up more. I had forgotten about the time on the clock. I had also forgotten that Joe had had a heart procedure about three weeks prior. What kind of jerk am I to tell him to sprint with me? But run he did and we shared a hand shake as I crossed the finish line – four seconds over 3:30.

Drat.

It is something to the mentality of a runner that they can wake up not even wanting to leave the bed and then be disappointed by a measly four seconds just a few hours later. But that is what racing is about. This ended up being one of my slowest marathons ever (131 of 146) but I have never been more proud of my effort. Throw in both the 165-mile run prior to it, a trip to Ecuador just three days prior to that, and a half marathon personal best the week before and I think I may have earned myself some rest.

Race: Leadville Marathon

Typical Date: Mid-June

Distance: Marathon

Location: Leadville, CO

Why You Should Run It:

Leadville is the highest incorporated city in the United States. Its population is 2,622. You know, like 26.22 miles in a marathon. Do you really need anything more to tell you that you should run this marathon? Well, I will be glad to share with you.

Cresting at 13,185 feet at Mosquito Pass the views will leave you breathless figuratively, if you're not already that way literally. The first two miles go up about a thousand feet. Then you drop 500 feet in a mile before climbing 1,200 feet in two more miles. Then you lose another 1,000 feet in two miles, pick up another 400 feet in a mile, lose 100 in the next mile before starting a 3.1-mile, 3,000-foot climb to Mosquito Pass. After that you just, more or less, repeat in the reverse to come back to home.

There are some races which you should do if for no reason other than bragging rights. This is one of them.

My Experience:

This race was the literal halfway point of my 52 marathons in 2006. I ran it again in 2012 and improved my time by over 45 minutes. However, it is the slower time from 2006 which will stick with me forever. I grew up at a measly 1,200 feet elevation in NW Pennsylvania.[156] When I ran this race I was living in Arlington, Virginia at 202 feet above sea level. It would be quite the understatement to mention I was hardly acclimated to run it when I got there. Throw in a major travel snafu even getting to

---

[156] To be honest, when I realized it was this high many years later, I was a little shocked. I always assumed we were at sea level.

the race, and let's say landing at midnight in Denver, two hours from Leadville, for a 7 a.m. start time is not how you want to take on a race which sits five times higher than you have ever been in your life.

I could bloviate about how grueling this race is and how the view from the top is mind-blowing but you can probably assume all of that from the above description. So allow me to tell you something you have likely never heard before from a race report.

If you know anything about running in the mountains it is wise to be prepared for any sort of weather. While we were mostly fortunate with regards to not getting hit by lightning or snow or anything else out of the blue, I was still wearing gloves just in case.[157]

Everything was going as well as I could expect it to when I came to that tortuous 3,000-foot climb to the top. I felt no shame in walking as virtually everyone had been reduced to a crawl here. Bent over at the waist, I was trying to force myself up the hill using every trick I could. As my legs were quite tired, I was relying on my arms to help with the load. I would push down on each quad with the corresponding hand when I stepped and repeated this ad infinitum. Place hand. Step. Push with hand as it slides down the leg. Repeat. This method actually assisted me a great deal in moving up the incline.

I crested the mountain, took a picture with the camera I had in my shorts pocket[158], and began the long trek home. It is a treacherous return with not only a screaming amount of downhill, but on uneven rocky footing with other people trying to get to where you just were. You can imagine all my concentration was on the task at hand.

---

[157] In a last-minute decision, I also purchased some black dress socks, cut the toe out of them and pulled them over my bare arms for some protection from the sun and potential elements. Nothing but style for this guy.

[158] Actually, I went to take a picture, started taking a video which meant I never took a picture and instead got a video of the inside of my shorts pocket and horrendous rustling sounds magnified by the camera's microphone until apparently my quadriceps turned the camera off on the decline somewhere.

When I finished in a time of 5:17:41, and in the top 50, I was one of only six people who did not live at some absurd elevation. I was ecstatic with how I had performed. Still on a high, I hurried to my lodging, stripped down to shower, and hopped in. Looking down I noticed the oddest thing ever. I am not a particularly hirsute chap but I do have a bit of hair on my legs. However, on each quad I had a one-inch thick strip the length of my quad that was absolute bereft of hair. Smooth as a baby's bottom and quite red, it looked like I had shaved a strip on my legs. Suddenly, I realized that with each sliding motion of my hands on my legs as I attempted to propel myself up the mountain, I had basically given myself a wax job.[159]

So, if you need to have some hair removed, and have about two hours to spare, I can gently, with a pair of dollar store cotton gloves, rhythmically remove a one-foot-long stretch of hair off your body, an inch-wide strip at a time.

---

[159] Ahhhhhh Kelly Clarkson!

Race: Niagara Falls Marathon

Typical Date: Second Sunday in October

Distance: Marathon

Location: Buffalo, NY and Niagara Falls, ON

Why You Should Run It:

Some races really are a no-brainer. Being able to run a marathon along the shores of the Niagara River, ending at one of the most iconic sights in all the world is one thing I barely have to sell you on. Adding to that the fact you get to cross an international border and also run a flat and fast race in weather conditions which are almost always conducive to good marathon times should be enough to convince anyone. Trust me when I say you need to run this race.

My Experience:

I would like to say that if this was not my first-ever sub-three-hour marathon I would still recommend it. In fact, I know that I would. But it will be hard for me to not get a little nostalgic for finally running a marathon with a time that started with a "2."

This was my 42nd marathon out of 52 in 2006. I had been getting steadily faster throughout the year and had already set a new personal best a few weeks prior with a 3:05. I had even paced the 3:10 group at the Des Moines Marathon which was a bit of chutzpah given I had only broken 3:10 on a handful of times prior to that day. But when you are hitting on all cylinders, you go with it.

I ran a vast majority of this race with a French-Canadian woman who told me that from her past experiences of running the event, the biggest obstacle would be what the wind was doing once you crossed the bride from Buffalo to Ontario and began the steady thirteen-mile run to the finish. Running almost directly in one direction for half the race, if the wind was in your face, it would be a challenge. Anything else would be a blessing. As we scampered off the ramp and began to head north, I will never forget the smile on her face as she looked at me and said: "No wind."

The rest of the race is a blur. I had a scant ninety second cushion to play with at the halfway point and mile after mile slowly ate away at that. It got to the point where I could no longer do math and I knew it was going to be close to go under three hours. With 10K to go I was fearful I might be slightly over. Hitting the 5K mark I figured maybe I had a shot. Even a mile to go left me uncertain as to what my time would be. Only with literally .1 to go, when we hit the thirteen-mile mark for the half marathoners, did I finally allow myself to celebrate. I crossed the mat in 2:59:48 and have rarely had a more exciting finish in my life. There really was no reason I should have been running this speed this late in the year of my marathons but here I was.

It is fun to do what you shouldn't be able to do.

Race: Kentucky Derby Marathon

Typical Date: Last Saturday in April

Distance: Marathon

Location: Louisville, KY

Why You Should Run It:

With regards to horse racing, 99.9% of us know nothing about it. Yet when every one of us passes a field of these equine beauties we will exclaim "Horsies!"[160] And every one of us cares at least a little about the Kentucky Derby. Akin to a week every four years in the Olympics when swimming or curling is suddenly the most interesting thing on the planet, for a few minutes each May, we all start talking about our height in hands, eating carrots whole, and binging on sugar cubes.[161] Whether it is for the spectacle of drunken, rich morons in fancy stupid hats or drunken less-rich morons with kegs and mullets in a grass infield, or we just really like to watch ponies run fast, the Derby speaks to all of us. Now imagine how cool it would be to be able to run on the famed dirt those same horses run! Now stop imagining it as there is no way in hell they are ever going to let plebeians run there.

If you think about it, you really don't actually wish to subject yourself to such an arduous workout. But when you run one of the races during the weekend's events, you do get to run on pavement on the infield of the inside of the Derby's stadium. That's almost as special.

Louisville is a city which has grown up drastically in the past two decades. With this growth the marathon has experienced a similar reconfiguration and consideration of what it is to its runners. It will never be a huge race but the crowd and organizers treat the runners as if they are one of the top five largest races in the

---

[160] You know I am right.
[161] No? Just me? Ok.

country. The course seems to change relatively frequently with the big hills in Iroquois Park coming at different times now than they did for me when I ran the marathon in 2009 and the half in 2012.

The weather in late April/early May when the race is held is fairly regularly decent even if I experienced an insanely hot day once year. But the truth of the matter is, forget the crowds, forget the weather, forget the organization: you get to run through Churchill Downs!

My Experience:

When I ran the marathon in 2009, pacing the 3:10 group, I was in the middle of eight marathons in seven weeks, including a personal best and a variety of other really great races. Suffice it to say I was in fantastic shape. Unfortunately, when I came to town, I rode in on a wave of unbearable heat and humidity as the race took place during the hottest Kentucky Derby Marathon weekend ever. The weather destroyed me and everyone else running the race.

By the thirteenth mile I had lost every single pace group member off the back. I was all alone. In spite of the weather, I had held it together until the 20th mile. Then a slow drain started. Three miles later it was a sieve and I was leaking energy. Miles went from 7:15 to ten minutes to fifteen minutes per mile. The only thing keeping me going was the fact I knew I needed to get to cold water soon. When I finished in 3:24:51, my 72nd slowest marathon ever, I ended a streak of twenty-four consecutive Boston Qualifying times. I also failed to run the exact time needed as a pace group leader for the first and only time.

When I ran the race three years later it was just one month after I ran the entire coast of Oregon (~355 miles) in one week. Going into the race, people asked me if I was recovered. Really, it depended on what your definition of that word happened to be. Was I limping? Nope. Was I able to run, cycle, swim and ambulate with no problem? Yep. Was there any lingering soreness in my legs? Absolutely. Could I run a 13.1-mile race? Shouldn't be a problem. But how fast I run it is where we get into the gray area of answering that initial question.

The real answer is "There is no way in the name of all that is sugary and good was I recovered". For seven days I ran 50 miles a day over undulating terrain and through wind and rain, stopping to talk to kids all along the way. I was exhausted. Mentally. Physically. Emotionally. Bereft of energy. But I would toe the line at the Derby Mini and find out where I was on my recovery without a doubt.[162]

The weather was cloudy and a tad humid but overall not too bad for racing. While I was mentally prepared to run a 1:45 or slower, each mile of this race kept surprising me. As we left the confines of downtown Louisville and headed toward Churchill Downs, my speed did not falter. Halfway through the race, I picked up the pace a bit. With three miles to go I saw I was definitely going to run far faster than I could have imagined. So after not knowing if I would even break two hours, now I was angry I had not saved enough in the tank to break 90 minutes. Funny how perspective changes everything.

As I began to chip away at the time, still cognizant of the fact that pushing too hard here would net probably nothing but a whole big basket of foolhardiness, I thought perhaps I could still break 1:31. Passing runners, I had time to think about how wonderfully organized the race was. The spectators were out in fair numbers and the water stations were plentiful. Moreover, the course was fast. After some changes from much tougher courses in the past, I was upset I wasn't in shape to race this course. One could run a VERY fast time here.

As I made the final turn and headed toward the home stretch, I saw I was going to break 1:31. Crossing the finish in 1:30:47, I would say I was more than pleased with how my body had responded. This race proved to me for the umpteenth time, in spite of the

---

[162] I really despise when races call their half marathon a "mini." I barely can stand the name "half marathon."

fact that I have Gilbert's Syndrome, for some odd reason, my body seems to respond best when it is racing a great deal. Go figure.

Race: Tucson Marathon

Typical Date: Second Saturday in December

Distance: Marathon

Location: Tucson, Arizona

Why You Should Run It:

An emphasis on downhill marathons has hit many races in the past few years. I personally feel that while downhills can obviously give you an edge, it is one you must take. You can't just coast downhill. We don't have wheels, after all. There is also a law of diminishing returns. Your quads will eventually buckle if you run too long on such a downward grade. You can learn how to do it better, and prep yourself for it, but it is by no means easy.

The Tucson Marathon has a forgiving downhill which is much more gradual than other downhill races out there. In addition, its place in the calendar means the weather is likely to be relatively cool, and since it is Tucson, quite dry. As it is exposed to the elements you run the risk of a long steady headwind as the course, for the most part, runs in one direction. But given that it has a little out-and-back with a surprise hill (if you haven't read this book) I think that all the pros of the race are evened out a bit making it one where you can run quite fast, but it will take a solid effort from you.

Plus you run by Biosphere. How cool is that?

My Experience:

I knew this race would be divided into three separate sections. The portion of mostly downhill from the beginning to the ten-mile mark would be the first. Going into this race I was hoping for a big personal best and was shooting for a 2:45:59. That would be a six-minute PR but it felt doable. Averaging out to around 6:20-miles, it was easy to do the math when I was running. Every three miles was equal to nineteen minutes.

I did my best to hold back at the beginning, even though I wanted to take advantage of the marvelous downhill start. Mile after mile felt perfect. So you can imagine when I hit the sixth mile in exactly 38 minutes, I was quite happy. I only had to do that for four more miles to finish this first section I had carved out in my mind. No need to worry about the remaining sixteen miles just yet. I wasn't there. At nine miles, I was exactly on pace at 56 minutes and finishing off the tenth mile in 1:03:30 I was only ten seconds off the goal – a mere rounding error.

The next section to contend with was the one near Biosphere. I had been warned there were some rolling hills on this out-and-back section. On the two-mile out section I lost a minute off my goal pace; half from the hills, half from me intentionally slowing to save myself for later. But after only losing another ten seconds heading back to the main highway, I was feeling pretty good. Now just twelve miles to go.[163]

Back on the highway, clouds overhead, dry weather all-around, it was perfect for me to run fast. My overall place did not matter to me but I felt I was in the top ten. With the long stretch of highway in front of us, I could see a few runners but I knew the distance between us was minutes, not seconds. I was focusing only on my time. If I could get to mile 20 feeling as good as I did, I felt I could run 6:40s and go sub 2:50. However, right at mile 20, the race changed.

A barely perceptible uphill rose beneath our feet and I could feel time begin to slip away. Each mile was slower than the next. Ten seconds lost here; twenty seconds lost there. I was aware there was a big hill at the 24th mile and was prepared to lose a little time there but wasn't expecting to do so now.

Unfortunately, that is exactly what happened. At mile 23, I ran my first seven-minute mile of the day and the hopes for a sub 2:50

---

[163] The "only" in this and how ridiculous the premise remains is not lost on me.

were more or less gone. The lead woman passed me with three miles to go. This was the first time since the beginning of the race that anyone had passed me. I figured I could stay with her and feed off her energy but she steadily pulled away.[164] My final good goal for the day was to do my best to try to get a new personal best, no matter how small the margin. But to be 100% honest, I did not care at this point to do so. This is a lousy attitude but it was the attitude I had. Plus, every single time I tried to push just a little bit, I felt like I might be bringing up some of the contents of my stomach. So, I just kept running. A runner passed me with about half a mile to go and I had no answer for him, either, even when he urged me to join him.

I could see the finish line ahead and the clock ticking away. All of a sudden the competitive juices began to flow. I picked up the pace as best I could, pushing forward all the way through to the finish line arch of balloons. I immediately doubled over, feeling like I was going to vomit.

This feeling passed just a few seconds later and as the announcer told the crowd about my 52 marathons I was quite happy I hadn't spilled my guts. Then I remembered my time! I quickly clicked my watch but did not know how long ago I crossed the line. When my results were not posted immediately, I went to the race results people. Apparently, my chip had not registered anywhere on the course.

Oh. My. God.

But before I could have a heart attack, they told me they would check the back-up timing mats. Sure enough, my time *did* register. 2:51:40. I set a new personal best by one second.

Not a bad day in Arizona.

---

[164] She eventually finished in 2:50:12 so if I could have stayed with her, maybe I could have broken in to the 2:40s.

Marathons and Relays

Race: Salt Flats 50K

Typical Date: End of April/Beginning of May

Distance: 50K

Location: Bonneville Salt Flats, UT

Why You Should Run It:

To run on the Bonneville Salt Flats. There really needs to be no other reason. If you don't recognize this place by its name, you have nonetheless seen them.[165] The Bonneville Salt Flats are one of the most unique natural features on Earth, stretching over 30,000 acres in Western Utah. Over the past century virtually every land speed record set has been done on these insanely flat, vegetation-less stretches of land. With a place devoid of any life, and so flat you can actually see the curvature of the Earth, you won't find a better place to start your race. If you can, that is.

What I mean by that ominous statement is because the very geography that formed these six-foot thick salt pans leaves it at the mercy of Mother Nature. The 50K is joined by a 50-mile race and 100-miler as well but only the first sixteen miles are on the flats.[166] After that, runners traipse off into the nearby mountains making this much more than just a speed race of flatness. However, after running the 50-mile race starting on the flats in 2015, both years I ran the 50K subsequently required some reconfiguring by the race crew.

Leading up to the race, rain storms blanketed the area leaving 50 square miles of a newly formed lake on the flats. As this new lake was just six inches deep, technically you could have run through it if your life depended on it. But fortunately, the race directors

---
[165] Have you seen the beginning of Knight Rider? Any car commercial ever? Pirates of the Caribbean Part 47? Well, then you have seen the flats!
[166] In fact, I take partial credit for the 50K even existing. When I ran the 50-miler I told the RD that it was an absolute shame that a simple out and back on the flats for a 50K didn't exist. The next year it did.

had a contingency plan which started runners in a different direction down the also very flat road leading away from the salt. Three-and-half miles of asphalt (or salt if you wanted to run next to the road) took racers out from the original starting point before heading off into the same mountain foothill trails runners would traverse later in the race in the longer distance events. Definitely more hilly, potentially more muddy, and requiring a little more lungwork than flat running, this out-and-back course shows how far the race directors are willing to go to make sure runners get their race. Nothing like having two completely different courses on hand for an entire slate of races, just in case.

My Experience:

My 50-mile race will be remembered for two main reasons: the fact I almost quit at the 50K mark, and getting lost around mile 42 or so. After a great start on the flats, the exposure to the elements got to me. By the time I got to the 50K aid station, I was completely encrusted in my own salt. In fact, I think the flats were jealous. I ambled into the aid station in second place but after well over a thirty-minute break, still wasn't sure I could go on. I finally decided, given the remoteness of where we were, it would have taken longer for someone to take me back to the start than it would be to simply finish the race. So I started running again.

After getting my carcass moving up a tough hill with some difficult footing and a rain storm out of nowhere, I was half-regretting the decision to continue. Ten miles later[167], when I found my groove and was cruising along dirt roads in the middle of nowhere, I passed right by a turn. Right as I reached the sign telling me to veer left, another runner's crew went by in a truck, obscuring the sign for just a split second. Turning my head to avoid the dust kicked up, I flat out missed the sign. A mile or so down the road I realized I was on the wrong course and had to double back. Adding distance to a race you wanted to quit is without a doubt the worst thing you can do. When I finally finished ninth overall

---

[167] Only in an ultra can you say "ten miles later" as if to say "well, nothing interesting enough to mention happened for an hour and a half."

I had a new personal worst in the 50-mile distance, but at least I had an official finish.

The following two years I ran the 50K, both times reveling in the fact that I had a hand in creating the course. And both times the rains came from nowhere and forced us to take the alternate route. We named it the Salt Flats Adjacent 50K. In the inaugural race in 2016, I set the course record by winning. Then I broke the record again in 2017. Unfortunately, so did another fella who cleaned my clock by 20 minutes relegating me to a second-place finish. Not too many races do you get to set and then break the course record in consecutive years and not win both times.

I was obviously disappointed to not be able to run on the flats portion for the 50K but the experience of doing so during the 50-mile was surreal. Rebar with flags attached to it is jammed into the salt to give runners guidance for running in a straight line. One would think simply running straight would be the easiest thing possible, but with no contextual clues to help you along, it is amazing how much you can drift off course. The island mountain out at the end of the flats[168] is tantalizingly close and also never seems to get any closer all at the same time. Suddenly, it is upon you and the flats are over. Luckily (in theory) those running the 50K get to run back over those flats again and see all the people behind them.

Without a doubt, the trailrunning community is populated with good people and when you are racing, it is both figuratively and literally nice to have them behind you.[169]

---

[168] Called this for the way the optical illusion makes it appear it is hovering over the ground in front of you.
[169] Because then you are beating many of them. Because it is a race. Forget it.

Race: JFK 50 Mile

Typical Date: Saturday before Thanksgiving

Distance: 50 mile

Location: Boonsboro, MD

Why You Should Run It:

The JFK began inauspiciously as one of a large number of "JFK Challenges" which sprung up in the winter of 1962-63. At the time President Kennedy challenged the U.S. Marines to see if they were fit enough to hike 50 miles in 20 hours, as Teddy Roosevelt's Marines had famously done. Unexpectedly, thousands of civilians took up the challenge as well.

Eleven men began the first JFK 50 Mile race. Four finished. Then JFK was assassinated.[170] Almost immediately most of these 50-mile challenges disappeared. But the JFK 50 Mile race in Maryland continued. And grew. In fact, it sells outs its 1,000 spots every year with some of the best running talent in the country toeing the line in Boonsboro, Maryland.

Unlike many trail races, JFK is much more runnable than one would think. Just not necessarily the Appalachian Trail section, though. Before you tackle this treacherous wooded trail, you run 2.3 miles on a typical road, where people run way faster than they should at the beginning of a 50-mile race. They do so because a bottleneck and conga line await them for the next half marathon or so on the Appalachian Trail. Expect some tough climbs and not the most discernible trail over roots and rocks and leaves once you enter here. Of course, with 1,000 people around you, chances are high you won't get lost. Once you leave the forest and you run a mismarked marathon distance[171] on the C&O Canal's crushed gravel surface along the Potomac River. The final portion of the

---
[170] Not, like, right at the race.
[171] Twenty-six point three.

race follows 8.4 miles of roads to Williamsport, Maryland.

All of this is run by a race director who was once a former course record-holder. Throw in the fact that it is run right around Thanksgiving and not only do you have a reason to wolf down turkey in a few days, but the weather in Maryland at the time is very conducive to running well. So, ask not what your quads can do for you…

My Experience:

I had one previous ultramarathon under my shoes when I toed the line for the JFK 50 Mile race. Two years previous I had taken on the Presque Isle Endurance Classic 12 Hour Run.[172] This race, however, was my final tune-up for running 52 marathons in 52 weekends, starting just six weeks after race day. My convoluted logic was that if I could run 50 miles in one setting, a hard-raced marathon every week for a year was possible. Why not?

I knew I wanted to get out of the gate fast and not get caught in the line of runners heading onto the Appalachian Trail. I did a decent job of doing just that as we plunged into a thicket of trees and leaves while still under the cover of a late fall morning darkness. Hiking the Appalachian Trail had been something I thought would be fun if I somehow ever had the time or resources. Running it here, I saw it would be an arduous task indeed, especially if most of it were as tough as this section was on the feet, knees, and quads.[173] I almost took a tumble on more than one occasion before fortunately righting myself. After each stumble, I would reallocate most of my resources to watching the person in front of me and stepping where they did in order to alleviate future missteps.

The first two miles are a tough climb, followed by a flat section of a mile and a half or so. Don't let the flat part fool you into thinking this section is easy. Beset with tons of twists and turns it will challenge you even if you aren't climbing. I remember thinking if I made it out of here without a broken ankle that, in and of itself,

---

[172] Discussed later in this book!
[173] Apparently, it is.

was a victory. The biggest climb of the race exploded in front of me as, in a mile's distance, I would ascend nearly six hundred feet. This is fortunately the highest you will get all day but you are not done with the hills just yet. For four miles I ran mostly downhill, loving the idea that any second I would pop out onto the C&O Canal. But when I started to climb again around nine miles in and did a series of ups and downs for the next five miles, I no longer knew what to believe.

Finally and mercifully, around mile 15 the screaming downhill to the canal's towpath began. Oodles of switchbacks at breakneck speed soon spit me out onto this crushed gravel. I knew this portion would be about as flat as one could hope for and set my sights on trying to make up distance on those in front of me. The next marathon distance was a challenging one on the mind in spite of the lack of elevation change. The course had a lulling sense to it which made it challenging to tell how far you had run. Occasionally, the path would straighten out but often you felt like were on a never-ending curve. With the woods omnipresent and the Potomac River always on the left, gauging distance can be task. I remember clearly being very excited when we finally left the towpath and got out onto the roads. The first big hill on those roads, almost immediately after leaving the towpath, sucked that happiness out of me.

For the next eight miles I thought about how I was pleased with whatever time and place I finished. This was all a setup for my big goal the next year and getting out of here unscathed was the biggest success. Coming in far slower than I expected but 97th overall (out of 952 finishers) was a heck of a feather in my cap. It gave me the confidence I needed to think that maybe I could just go do something I was continually being told was impossible.

Race: Iron Horse 50 Mile

Typical Date: Second Saturday in February

Distance: 50 miles

Location: Florahome, FL

Why You Should Run It:

When I ran this race it consisted of a short out-and-back to the west for a total of three miles before heading back east for eleven miles. Runners would then turn around to complete one 25-mile loop at the starting line before heading out again for the second loop. It doesn't get much simpler than that when it comes to direction. In spite of the simplicity, there was an extremely challenging portion which, as the great Monty Python once said, was covered in "very small rocks." Well, the small rocks section has since been paved over which is exceedingly wonderful for all of you reading this as that makes it infinitely easier. The absolute straight left and then right running has changed a touch as well. They have added an additional lollipop loop and another out-and-back off of the main trail to contend with. So while those have changed, it remains virtually the same in spirit.

There are crew points at about five spots on the course which allows easy access for those who are there to support you. In fact, for long stretches of the race your crew is just a stone's throw away through the bushes onto a nearby road. In addition, there are three manned aid stations stocked with food and drink. With weather in northern Florida often being much chillier than most imagine for February, conditions are ripe for an excellent time. In other words, if you are looking to tackle your first ultramarathon over the 50K distance, this race should be one you absolutely consider.

My Experience:

The weather for my Iron Horse 50 Mile race (partly cloudy skies, cool temperatures and low humidity) was amazing. Not unlike the weather I had the previous week at another 50-mile race where I had to cut short because of lingering flu symptoms, I was ecstatic. Rarely does training, weather, and course awesomeness all come together like that. For it to happen twice in two weeks was actually a little nerve-wracking. In my mind, I HAD to do well here as who knew when I would get the perfect confluence again.

Friday night before the race called for a race briefing by race director Chris Rodatz, who provided humor and directions to the runners in attendance. We got to learn a little bit more about the course and had our interest piqued about a few areas. The one thing which grabbed my attention the most was the old railroad trestles on this rails-to-trails course. Rotting and ancient, they required Chris himself to nail down wooden 2x4s side-to-side to create a planked road for runners to traverse. His description painted a picture not unlike the various rope bridges we have seen in Indiana Jones movies.

I had attended this meeting, and later dinner, with my friend Kelly Luckett and her husband. Kelly, an amputee runner, was attempting her first 50-mile race, in an effort to be one of the first with a prosthetic leg to ever do so. Her pluck and determination were both inspiring and admirable. When we parted ways for the night, I had visions of both of us conquering this 50-mile beast.

Unfortunately, I could not fall asleep. Nerves, typical restlessness, or whatever else kept me up until 1:30 a.m. With a wake-up call at 4:30 to accompany Kelly and her husband[174] on the 40-minute drive from our hotels in Orange Park to the race start in Florahome, these three hours of sleep were not nearly the amount I was hoping to get.

I used the aid stations as five separate points to break the race down into smaller parts in order to make it more manageable in my mind. With so much math going on in my head, I really just wanted to get going. When we lurched out of the gate at 7 a.m., it

---

[174] Brian would run with Kelly for the entirety of the race which was a very challenging feat given his 3:40 marathon PR and their projected pace of much slower than that. Running slow is hard. No joke here.

was a huge relief just to be running.

A few yards into the race, two runners took off in front of me. Upon speaking with them, I found they were both running the 100K, so their effort meant nothing to me. Nevertheless, when they began to pull away, I was intrigued to see if they would keep that pace for the whole race.

As we completed the first turnaround, marked with signs that said "T/R"[175] I could see I had more than a slight lead on just about every other runner out there. Another man had slipped past me in this first little bit but he too was running the 100K. It was a bit odd to be in fourth place overall when all three of the guys were supposedly running longer than me.

Hitting the starting point again, I shed my outer layer and now was into a groove with just a singlet and a t-shirt underneath. Still waking up, I was ready to see what the course had in store for me. We had already crossed one of the aforementioned railroad trestles after a few more miles and while they did not provide the best footing available, they were not the death traps some of us had feared. We now settled into running on what would be the remainder of the course— hard-packed dirt and pine needles with large-stoned gravel intermittently dispersed underfoot.

For the most part this footing was adequate, but the stones were indeed large enough to twist an ankle or provide enough rolling to leave one sore afterward. Poor Kelly twice hit the dirt when her prosthetic running foot caught the gravel. But even with a bloodied knee she ventured forth, like a freaking rock star.

I hit a Porta-Potty at the second aid station on the course and upon emerging finally felt both awake and good, as if I might actually do well. Until then, I was still unsure what would happen. The next stretch was spent simply looking at one of the 100K runners in front of me, never getting any further away but never getting any closer either. I wondered if I was too slow, he too fast, or a combination of both.

---

[175] Which I learned is Southern for "Turn 'Round".

Nearing the turnaround at the end I was shocked to see that the two lead 100K guys had not slowed and if anything were picking up the pace. I was able to catch the third 100K runner in front of me when I ran across the longest of the trestles and he walked. However, as he did not stop at the aid station and I did, he passed me again.

I was happy to have made up a little time on this short out-and-back in between the furthest aid station as my overall pace was off what I was hoping to run for the day. I would lose a little more time on what would be the longest stretch between aid stations for the day (just a touch over five miles) but overall was right on track. So plentiful and frequent were these aid stations that I did not even bother to carry any food or drink with me. I was feeling good, sharing pleasantries with the other runners as we passed in different directions, and could hardly believe I was already 18-plus miles into this race.

Hitting the last aid station before completing the first loop, I could see I was getting back on track time-wise for my goal. I knew my time was not nearly as important as the completion, but when you are leading a race, it is hard to shake those thoughts of winning.

As we neared the end of the first loop, I noticed the temperatures had not picked up very much, the sky was still cloudy, and the air was still cool and low in humidity. This gave me delusions of a negative split, which are fairly uncommon in a 50-mile race. My time of 3:17:04 at the halfway point put me just a touch off my desired goal of running a 6:30 overall 50 mile time.[176]

Having passed the third 100K runner when he stopped to walk at mile 20, I was now in no man's land. As far as I could see in front of me there were no runners to chase. And believe me, you could see forever. The blue tents marking the aid stations would appear on the horizon and then ten minutes later you still would not have reached them. As such, I did my best to just use the 100K runners in front of me to pace myself if they ever appeared. After a stellar

---

[176] That's a 7:48 minute mile for those of you scoring at home. Or even if you are alone.

beginning three-mile loop to kick off the second 25-mile section, I knew I was closing in on them.

I may have pushed this beginning portion a little too hard as soon I felt a slowing in my legs. I tried to tell myself I just had an approximate 30-minute run, followed by a 40-minute run, which then led into a 20-minute run, before I only had a 40-minute run which would allow me to end with a 30-minute run. Somehow this seemed comforting. Yet, when I got to the aid station two-plus minutes behind my goal, I was a little bummed. I had caught one of the remaining 100K runners in front of me. He was not looking good. With his hands on his knees, not taking in any food or drink, he seemed done for the day. As I left the area, I felt a bit of speed slip back into my legs.

Unfortunately, now I knew I would be running solo again. The 100K runner leading this race was simply not in sight and with runners who were way behind me coming at me in the opposite direction it was hard to gauge my speed. At the aid station before the turnaround, however, my watch told me the slowing process was continuing. Arriving five minutes slower than I had on the previous loop, this section had taken much more out of me than I wanted to give.

Seeing the lead runner not so far ahead at least helped my ego a bit. I was quite amazed at the pace he was holding and was extremely pleased he was running the 100K. Then I recalled runners had the option of dropping down from one distance to another at any time. My previous laissez-faire attitude spilled out of me. I had to make up ground on him! And make up ground I did on the next little section but at too much of a cost. With nine miles left in my race, I knew I was most definitely paying for my quickened pace. If he dropped down to the 50-mile distance, and I ended up in second place, so be it.

The sun had finally come out and when it flitted in between the branches it was a welcome feeling. I was not generating the same amount of heat as normal. My core temp had dropped a bit and I was more than ready to be finished. I wanted to sit down and put on something warm and comfortable. I blazed through the last aid station and found the 100K runner was just a few minutes in front of me.

My energy was definitely fading. With both a sub-6:30 and sub-6:40 time out of reach, I would walk a few steps here and there. The gravel had definitely gotten the better of me a few times and my ankles, more specifically my right one, were aching. When I saw Kelly up ahead nearing the completion of her first loop, I welcomed the opportunity to walk with her a bit on one of her breaks.

She was in good spirits for sure, even if she was more tired and slightly further behind than she had hoped to be. I minded not one bit the break here as I knew I was miles ahead of the next competitor. We walked together and she told me how she had fallen and how hard it was for her to find any consistency with running because of the footing. I listened and commiserated the best I could. Finally, after a while, my legs wanting to be done spurred me forward into running again.

As I hit the final hundred yards, I realized how tense and nervous I had been all day. Now here I was, not only completing the course but leading it wire-to-wire. I had no one to run with, no one to pace with, and virtually no one to chase. The nagging feeling of tiredness which crept in, inevitably and understandably on the second loop, would not normally have given me pause. But after the DNF of the previous weekend, it was hard to establish if it was normal tired or soon-to-be-stopping-with-no-energy tired. However, a few minutes later, I was crossing the finish line, taking first place and breaking the course record by 50 minutes.

Unfortunately, Kelly finally succumbed to both exhaustion and the rapidly-dipping temperatures and had to pull out at mile 46. She simply could not keep her core temperature up in the chill of the night and wisely stopped before anything permanent was done to her system. Nevertheless, I was blown away by her effort. You needn't have obvious reminders like Kelly's disability to make sure you don't take what you have for granted. However, when you see what can be done by those who have "less" it is a vivid reminder to do the best you can every day with what you have.

Race: Sawtooth Relay

Typical Date: Sunday before Memorial Day

Distance: 61.9

Location: Stanley to Ketchum, ID

Why You Should Run It:

Perhaps you are looking to do a relay but not wishing to take on something of the all-day variety. You crave the camaraderie which is intermingled with running with teammates but would prefer not to run three runs in one day. While long-distance relays are popping up everywhere, there is something to be said about running a little shorter and a little faster. If you can do so in one of the surprising hidden gems of beauty in America, then that's even better.

It is hard for much of anything to stay too hidden anymore in today's world of social media and a camera attached to everything. Heck even this book is a camera. Look on the back![177] But somehow the pristine gorgeousness that is Idaho's Sawtooth National Forest remains relatively off the radar for most people. Long the playground of the Hollywood elite during their ski trips, there is no reason why runners should not be able to treat themselves as well to this majestic and beautiful area.

As the race does a 25-mile slow gradual climb from Stanley, Idaho before shooting up 1,500 feet in five miles, you can imagine your view will change tremendously. The second half's elevation chart looks like a mirror image of the first half as you run down the other side of Galena Summit toward Ketchum. From babbling brooks to wide open high plains, only the rugged and aptly named Sawtooth Mountains in the background are able to compete with the rest of the scenery for pure effervescence. As the entirety of the race is run on pavement, this is not a technical or challenging

---

[177] Please tell me you didn't look.

race, either logistically or footing-wise. Basically, you get on one road and head south until you turn off into a park and are done. But what you lack in turns you make up for in visual splendor.

My Experience:

I took on this race as a solo participant. Initially I thought I might need to convince the race directors to allow me to do so but upon reviewing the website found there was a solo division. On race day, however, I was just one of three taking on the course alone.

My biggest fear on race day was the potential for heat and sunlight. The entirety of the race course would be run out in the open with no tree cover to mention. I have well-documented my struggles with running in the heat and am greatly jealous of those who handle it far better than I do. Yet, as the day approached, the entire area was dealing with unprecedented chilly and rainy weather.

So now my fears went from heat and how to deal with that to how I was going to stay dry and non-chafed through nearly 100K of running.[178] I had given thoughts to running the race unassisted but rules stipulated I needed a support crew. A friend in Idaho mentioned she had a co-worker who was always up for adventure and would ask to see if she would wish to crew for me. Presto change-o, Jessica and her sister Melody became my two-person crew! Now all I had to do was run 62 miles, in the rain, topping out at 8,701 feet, by myself.

Based on the time I thought it would take me to finish, I was given a 4 a.m. start.[179] Yuck. Double yuck when that calls for a 3 a.m. wake-up call. You get the triumvirate of yuck when, try as you might, you cannot fall asleep until after 1 a.m. Oh well, two hours of sleep should be enough, right?[180]

---

[178] "Nearly" because the race is 61.9 miles. I had lobbied the RD to add .2 so it would be a true 100k but to no avail.

[179] Teams are sent out at certain times to maximize the potential of most teams finishing around the same time. Ergo, slower teams start first.

[180] Right?!

There were twelve legs of this course and even though I was running alone, if I broke them down as such it almost didn't seem so bad. Even more, I chopped it into three distinct races: the long, gradual uphill to the mountain at the middle of the course, up and down that mountain; and then the long, gradual downhill to the finish.

The first 27 miles until I began the ascent to Mt. Galena were very similar. A general weirdness pervaded my senses as I ran on the right-hand side of the road, which goes against the nature of a runner. Yet that was where the exchanges and aid stations were and the rules stipulated we stay there, so suck up the weirdness, Dane

After the first few legs were done, the sun began to tickle the darkness out of the night sky and hints of the mountains began to develop in the distance. I was eagerly anticipating what beauty the daylight would bring. I thought as the day wore on I might need to change to a short sleeve shirt but the weather stayed cool for longer than expected. In fact, before long, it started to drizzle. It never poured but rather the rain hung in the air just long enough to wet clothing. For the most part, this rain wasn't a problem for everyone else just running six miles. Regardless, after a marathon of running, the summit erupted in front of me.

It became quite clear there would be points where powerwalking would be just as fast as running as I began the 1,331-foot climb to Galena Summit. When I would pass someone or get passed, I would always have the same exchange: "What bet did you lose to get this portion of the course?" It always got a laugh. Misery, company, something something.

As I continued to climb, and in spite of the rain, I felt surprisingly warm. My assumption was as I approached 9,000, I would feel a chill. Heck, there was still plenty of snow on the cliff walls around me. Then I realized the rain had stopped and my body temperature was finally rising. The temperature never topped 50 degrees for the first half of the race, but I felt once I crested the summit and headed toward the finish in Ketchum, things would change.

Running the backside of Galena Summit with its 1,401 feet of downhill did not provide the warmth I thought. Once again I felt a nip in the air. I flagged down my crew and asked for my heavier jacket. This part of the race marked where I finally began passing fewer runners and began getting passed by more. The attrition of the race was taking over as fresher runners running shorter distances were gaining on me.

Unfortunately, the superb weather I assumed might await me on the other side of the mountain never materialized. Instead, I was getting soaked. My routine became one of me handing over a drenched outer layer to the girls who would put it across the heater of the car and hand me a dry shirt. Then, at the next exchange, we would change from the shirt I had on to the one from the vehicle. The siren's song of the exchange stations became harder to ignore. I would sit down to grab some calories and then would have the hardest time moving along again. You will hear ultraunners often say "Beware the chair"[181] but the truth remains I needed every break I took.

The last thirteen miles became more time spent in the chair in between legs and an overall slowing of pace, which was to be expected. What was unexpected was what happened about half way through the penultimate leg. As I began to gain ground on one particular runner I decided to take a small walk break. When I began running again, he had gone around a curve. Once I was able to make a visual on him again, I saw he was crossing the road. He hopped into a van and another male teammate began running in his place. As we were running the same pace I could not make up any ground to ask what the hell they were doing. About a mile later, again around a turn, I saw this replacement runner hop into the same van and then a woman appeared where he had been. I was completely stunned. Were they really cheating in leg 11 of a race where it was quite obvious they would be finishing in the bottom third? Then I thought that perhaps this was allowed. I never got an answer to my question as they were able to separate from me. At the very least they kept me thinking about something else for a while.

---

[181] Mostly because it rhymes.

With two miles to go, every single cloud evaporated from the sky like someone had turned on a vacuum. The rain stopped, the sun beat down, and I laughed out loud. How could it go from nine-and-a-half hours of crappy weather to a beautiful day so suddenly? Regardless, I found myself quite spent. Running along a bike path, the small but abrupt undulations brought me to a slow walk every time. Four or five teams passed me in these final miles and most I recognized as teams that had started at the same time as I had about ten hours earlier. I was bummed I had not been able to hold them off but was elated to be done. Entering Atkinson Park I could hear a band playing in the distance. Some helpful volunteers guided me across the street and stopped traffic.

10 hours, 36 minutes and 59 seconds after the odyssey began it was done. I won the solo race and beat my fair share of teams as well, with 70 of the 290 teams finishing behind me. Yet even if I had finished dead last, I would still recommend you head to this relay in central Idaho.

But bring teammates.

Race: River to River Relay

Typical Date: Middle Saturday in April

Distance: 80 miles

Location: Southern Illinois

Why You Should Run It:

A main reason to run this race is to challenge yourself in a not-so-talked-about locale. When the repetitive lists which caused me to write this book tell you which places to run, you can bet your bottom dollar they are not mentioning southern Illinois. They should. And if you are lucky enough to get into this venerable relay (the 250 spots fill in about five *minutes*), consider it both a blessing and a curse. It's a blessing because the race is entering its fourth decade and is finely-tuned from soup to nuts. It's a curse mostly if you are the runner to draw the third-to-last leg, a brutal climb that brings many to a crawl.

Otherwise, set in bucolic part of the country, this 80-mile relay is just the sort of event for runners looking to take on the relay experience but not wanting to spend 24-26 hours to accomplish that. Since most participants will not do more than ten miles total over three separate legs, virtually anyone who can complete a 5K can be part of a team.

My Experience:

Or, if you have a buddy who likes to really run long like you do, a little schmoozing with the race director can make you and this buddy the only two-man team to ever take on the race. Unfortunately for my friend, a prior active-duty Marine, Mosi Smith, and I, the mid-April temperatures soared. Originally projected for a high of 76, still too hot for my tastes, we had a mid-day scorcher of 86 instead. Then again, Mosi likes the heat, having completed the Marathon De Sables and Badwater races. Regardless, it was going to be a hard day for Team Ebony and Ivory.[182]

As I drove and did not run Mosi's portions of the race, it is hard for me to comment on them specifically. I do know that according to Mosi and the website, there were no three consecutive runs which rated "easier" than his first of the day. Throw in the fact that these were run in the morning, when the temperature was still 55 degrees, as well as mostly in the shade, and Mosi had it made. This is verified by the fact he was cruising along at barely over seven minutes per mile. I told him before we started to take it easy. He needed to remember we were each running 40 miles that day.[183]

I took off on my first set of legs knowing it would require me to run a few miles until I felt good. Let's just say that not everything on the ole body had been working well. Not with the broken hand at Christmas a few months before and the 103-degree pneumonia in March. Naturally, I started my run and immediately went up a hill. Not a big one but a hill nonetheless. Soon thereafter, someone passed me. Our rule for the day was it didn't matter who passed us. We had to remember that virtually everyone else was running ten miles total, as most teams had at least eight members to their team. Yet when you are a competitor it is one thing to say you should think this way. It is another thing entirely to follow through with sane, rational plans.

Before long, I caught the gentleman who passed me and said "good job" to him. Then the course sloped down a bit and I finally felt half-decent. Soon thereafter, we reached the first exchange and that same runner sprinted past me to hand off. I casually ran through the relay and began my second leg. I doubted that would be the last time that would happen all day. I also didn't realize this would be my easiest run of the entire race.

The next two legs presented quite a bit more hills. But I was still fresh and it wasn't too hot. Yet. I ran with a few people whose teams I would see a great deal of throughout the day. In fact, the 6:20 Club Team pulled up to me and said; "Hey, we are behind you

---

[182] Yep, we had it on the side of our vehicle.
[183] He didn't listen to me.

and are a team of eight. Can you please slow down?" I laughed and said if they would carry my water I would think about it.

I crested the last little hill, handed the baton to Mosi, and he handed the car keys to me. We were 25% done for the day.

Between both dropping Mosi off the first time and here, I got caught in a bit of a bottleneck of cars. When you have a team, a bottleneck doesn't add too much stress to everyone. When you are the only other driver and runner, little setbacks like this are far worse. As it was, I barely made it to park before Mosi was on me.[184]

I was happy to know that this leg was a little shorter than my first one. There were also no hills. Well, I take that back. The River to River Relay is virtually nothing but hills. In fact, there are few times when you are on a flat. So it all comes down to a matter of perspective. In this instance, there were no hills that I audibly groaned at when I saw them.[185]

This section, however, was where I was 100% exposed to the elements. With a bright hot sun overhead, and running on open roads, I could tell I was slowing more than I would like. I was trying to focus on just getting to the exchange but then I realized that Mosi's next run would be his shortest of the legs all day. It would also be the easiest. This meant I would have even less time than normal to rest and recover. I shouldn't have thought that far ahead but when you have to plan and conserve, there are many factors you must consider.

In my first two legs I passed double-digit runners. I tried my best to encourage them all. Unfortunately, some had headphones in and I didn't want to waste my energy if they couldn't hear me. So I would often just give a thumbs up as I passed, hoping it was encouraging to them. At the same time, I hoped, out of the corner of their eye, they did not think I was giving them the bird.

<u>As Mosi began</u> his third set of legs the temperature climbed

[184] Not literally. I mean, we are buddies and everything but geesh.
[185] I may have still let out a slight whine.

dramatically and his pace did as well. If we had been able to communicate (cell reception was all but non-existent) and had a third person to handle driving duties, it might have been wise to break up the legs differently. Unfortunately, all we had was our feet to get us to the next exchange.

I had a relatively smooth going through to get to next stop. When Mosi came in, we exchanged our normal pleasantries to tell each other how we felt, where the car was, etc. He then told me he was baked from the sun. Knowing it was getting hotter and Mosi runs in heat better than I do was not a good feeling.

I did the math and could see that unless we had a herculean effort in both of our last legs, we probably were not going to break ten hours like we had wanted. But if we were able to keep everything in check then sub-eleven was no problem.

My first portion of this next section went fine. Not great but fine. Every once in a while a runner from another team might catch me and chat for a bit. I wanted to be friendly but I also wanted to save my energy. It is hard to do both. The second portion of this leg was just about the same. Slower pace, friendly runners. Then when I began the last portion I began to feel the heat. I felt like what Mosi had described at the end of his last leg. With two miles left in this leg I took a quick walking break and drank heartily from my Camelbak. This seemed to help and I powered forward. With one mile left, I knew I needed to take another walking break. As I took this break and made a turn I was presented with a rather cruel uphill. As I began moving, my legs seized up. I came to a dead stop.

I was offered water by one runner and more from another. I knew, however, that lack of water was not the problem. It was a complete lack of salt that I had tried to balance throughout the race. I had the energy. I could powerwalk. But if I tried to run, searing pain shot through the entire quad like lightning. I knew that stopping here wasn't an option. I had to suck it up, walk, and hopefully get ready for my last three legs.

As I approached the handoff I told Mosi what had happened. I asked him if he thought he could pick up one of my legs for me. Instead of him doing three and me three, if he could do two and then I did one and we repeated that, we could finish this. I knew he was tired but I also knew at this point I couldn't do what we needed to do. It is one of the things I have learned about my body from having Gilbert's Syndrome. Once I am wrecked, there is almost no coming back from it without serious time off and calories in. He said he could do it. I can't tell you how grateful I was for that.

With just two legs to get ahead, I knew this was going to be even tighter than normal for me to get to the exchange. As I passed Mosi while driving I told him to simply go slow. It would allow me to recuperate and would keep him from hurting himself as well. As it had been a 41.85 to 38.15 mile split with our original plan in my favor, I told him this would also give him bragging rights as the numbers would be reversed. He smiled his million-watt smile and away I went.

When I parked and began walking I knew I had a blister on my toe. But I didn't have time to take care of it at this point. Plus I knew I needed to walk around and get ready for my next leg. The last thing I needed to do to Mosi was not be ready.

When he rolled into the exchange, I knew something was not good. He told me he simply could not do the extra leg. I know Mosi and if there is any way he can push himself to do something, he will do it. If he said no, then it was a definite. The only problem was that I had only brought my handheld from the car and not my normal Camelbak. It was too far to go back, and I didn't have the energy to add extra miles. I told him he had to go to the next exchange and meet me there with the car and liquid. I couldn't do two legs with just the handheld. I didn't realize how right I was.

Without a doubt I was a bit crestfallen I had to do these two legs. There was no fault or blame put on Mosi; I had just convinced myself of what I could do. As I began the first portion, I could only run a bit before my legs threatened to cramp. The next three miles were much of the same. Awful tiredness, potential cramps, followed by my loathing of the situation. Anger welled up inside of me that we had made it so far doing so well just to have the end of the race completed in this death march.

Mosi was waiting for me with ice-cold water. I told him I needed to sit down in the car. While there, my friend David from Evansville, Indiana just a few hours away, stopped by the car to offer support. He too was taking on the leg that I was about to try to get through. I asked him what his take was on this next section and he paused. He looked like he didn't want to tell me what he had to tell me. "Um, it is the hardest leg of the entire course." Well, crap. To put it in the words of the race itself "This is the favorite section for everyone except Runner Number 6."

It was not pretty. It wasn't even ugly. Heck, I wouldn't even try to set this leg up on a date with my friends by saying it had a nice personality. I sheepishly trotted down the long downhill to start before crossing the bridge and seeing the hill from hell. Starting at 379 feet and going to 729 feet there was nothing to like. I walked virtually every step of this. My heart was lifted only by the fact that many of the runners in front of me didn't seem to be going all that much faster. Only pride pushed me forward in the last few yards to give the baton to Mosi.

Screw that jerky jerkface with his jerky being done jerkness. Oh yeah, he finished strong, too. Or something.

With just one leg to recover, there was no recovery. I had just given Mosi an hour and a half to recover and now I knew I wasn't going to get a third of that back. When I parked the car, I simply put the seat back and tried to get myself settled. Everything was cramping. My heart was racing. I looked at my shorts and saw they were covered in salt. My intention had been to change shorts throughout the day to keep them fresh but simply hadn't had the time to do so. However, I was slightly confused as I knew I had been wearing pure black shorts. When I brushed my leg with my hand, one of the odd patterns on the fabric brushed right off. I could have met the tequila-shot-drinking needs of an entire

Spring Break crew doing shots with the salt that came off me with one swipe.

Sitting there, I had zero desire to do this last 3.3 miles. I looked at the chart. Oh, good. It is a "hard" leg, too. Then I looked in the rear view mirror. There was Mosi. Only like seven hours earlier than I wanted him to appear.

I ambled out of the car, gave him a quick high-five as he gave me the baton and a swat on the ass. I then promptly shuffled out of the exchange zone. I couldn't run. I wanted to. For all the people who were cheering me on, I wanted to. I just couldn't.

I saw we had an hour and 45 minutes to finish the race under the time limit. I figured even if I crawled the last three miles that would still be enough. As before, I had energy, not much of it, but it was the cramping that was the problem. Again, I do not wish to bore you with the woe-is-me portion of this run, so I will simply skip ahead to the last mile where I could finally run again. Well, "jog."

As I approached the merciful end of this relay in Golconda, I could see Mosi waiting for me to run the last .2 of a mile. I told him that would still keep him two miles less than me for the day and I hated him and he was a poophead.

We trotted down the final stretch to more than a few cheers from the teams who had finished. Many I recognized from the run and had passed us in our last ten miles. I was a little ashamed to be ambling in after such a solid effort earlier in the day but the fact I was upright was an accomplishment in itself. As we neared the finish, I could hear another team coming up behind us. I looked at Mosi and said "There is no way in hell I am letting them pass me." I hobbled forward at double time and held off what was undoubtedly a great group of people who I had no intention of finishing after.

We held the baton aloft together, took a few steps, and crossed the finish line. I stopped my watch, and then embraced Mosi in a hug. Eleven hours and 48 minutes after we started, we could finally sit down.

Well, not just yet as a line of well-wishers had gathered. The last thing I wanted to do was seem rude to those who had stopped by to wish us congratulations. But I also thought it would be rude if I pitched forward as I passed out from exhaustion. So after a few conversations, I excused myself and sat down. Mosi, who doesn't exactly like the limelight, was forced into being the spokesperson for a bit. Thankfully, he had his wits about him a tad more than I did at this point.

Within a few minutes I was able to get moving again, albeit slowly. We spoke to the race director, Brad Dillard, and told him what a wonderfully put together race he had with excellent volunteers and staff. Virtually every runner we encountered was affable and friendly, whether they knew we were a two-man team or not. It is no secret why this race completely fills, year in and year out.

We were sincerely grateful to Brad for allowing us to compete as a two-man team as we knew he often gets such requests. I think, like all things in life, he looked at the totality of the circumstances and decided this one time would be worth the exception. We can only hope that we made everyone comfortable with their decision.

Ending mileage total: Mosi - 38.15; Dane - 41.85.[186]

---

[186] Not that anyone's counting.

Race: Presque Isle Endurance Classic

Typical Date: Mid-October

Distance: 12-Hour Timed Race

Location: Erie, PA

Why You Should Run It:

As running races grow and evolve in a variety of ways, many pop up which harken back to where racing was a century ago. Events where runners took on the clock to see how far they could run in a set time, rather than a set distance, were once races people flocked to see. It is hard to fathom now but jam- packed, smoked-filled stadiums once dominated the running scene. Often just following two or three runners around a tiny indoor track, men in top hats and suits would wager enormous sums of money on how much further one man could run than another.[187] Time passed and these events fell out of favor, as did running as a whole as the nation's first real pastime. However, these types of events are making a huge comeback. It's about time.[188]

This particular race was created over thirty years ago by a local running club in Erie and truly allows runners to test their limits in a great location. Situated on the peninsula which juts out into Lake Erie, and runs around a one-mile, pancake-flat loop under a thick shade of trees, the PIEC gives runners a chance to run for any period of time they wish within the 6:30 a.m. to 6:30 p.m. time frame.

With a mostly-paved route nestled in a thicket of wilderness, the race offers both the excellent footing of a road race but the feel of a trail race. Moreover, with an aid station every mile[189], there is

---

[187] Undoubtedly there was lots of "Chaps" and "Cheery-O!"s.
[188] I'll show myself out.
[189] Or a 1989 Ford Probe with cheese crackers, grapes, and Mountain Dew in the trunk, as was the case for me.

never a need to know where your sustenance is or how far until you can break. While the event states it is a personal thing and not one of competition, the simple fact remains that they are keeping count of how far you run; so as far as I am concerned, you are competing against someone.

My Experience:

I tackled this just one month after my second marathon ever. I was very much a neophyte in the running world and while 2003 wasn't the dark ages, it was well before any sort of social media. My knowledge of how to run an event such as this was absolutely nil. In fact, when I went through the first twenty-six miles only five minutes slower than my then-marathon PR, I figured I was doing a good job of pacing. What I did not know was that this might end up being my greatest running achievement ever.

With weather nearly perfect for me (cloudy, chilly and a little bit rainy) I was able to churn out mile after mile. Ignorance truly was bliss as there was no earthly reason for me to be running as well as I was on that day. When my miles piled up, someone decided to tell me the furthest anyone had ever run for the race. Doing the calculations, I felt I might just be able to best that and maybe a little bit longer. What I didn't know was no one had come close to that distance in over two decades.

As thirty miles turned into forty which then turned into fifty, I simply churned away. I had an mp3 player which held a little over an hour's worth of music. In fact, I still have this relic in a box somewhere. It was powered by one AAA battery and I could get about four listens out of it before it was dead. While I will, on occasion, listen to music in a long race, this event was where my first distaste for doing so started. I knew, at my pace, every song equaled about half a mile run. I then would start breaking it down further and further until I knew that one "Pour Some Sugar on Me" chorus equaled about 100 yards.[190] I never made it through the whole battery. After three times through, I took the headphones out and never put them back in.

---

[190] Ooh, in the name of love.

This race was the first taste I had of tying philanthropy to running. At the time I was a law clerk in Erie and had hit up many of my co-workers to donate on a per mile basis to the American Cancer Society. I had already lost a few members of my family to the disease and my grandfather was currently suffering from it as well. I will admit that I completely undersold how far I thought I could run but not intentionally. As I clocked mile after mile, I thought of how much money I was raising and it warmed my soul. I would lose my grandfather just a few months later but whenever I think of this race I think of him.

Runners were given a long plastic card that they had to keep safety-pinned to their clothing. Every mile you had to stop and have volunteers punch it with a special hole punch. I remember thinking that this was a horrible idea as it killed your momentum and then forced you to start again, often when you didn't have the gumption to do so. About halfway through the race, the rain picked up just enough that the volunteers moved into a cabin that housed all sorts of goodies and, more importantly, a warm fire. They told runners they would simply keep track of every lap you ran as you went by and when you came in they would punch your card. I think this is what gave me the spark I needed. I began coming into the cabin every four or five miles and taking as few breaks as possible. I felt like I was in so much more of a rhythm and zoned out for almost half an hour at a time. I began to name the Presidents. Then the Vice Presidents. Then the states and their capitals. I was in my happy place.

With about two hours to go, I could see the course record was mine for the taking. I thought grabbing that would be worth some local bragging rights but other than that didn't put much more of an emphasis on it. Even if I had known the last man to break the record had been in nineteen-eighty-something, I know I would have only thought it was some little record set in some little race tucked in the corner of northwestern Pennsylvania. I didn't know then that some of the most prestigious races often taken place in remote parts of the country.

A co-worker came down and I walked a mile or two with him. I knew I was going to break the record and I just didn't have the energy to run. But walking I could do. Soon thereafter and with no fanfare, I was told I broke the record and had nine minutes left in the 12-hour period. I figured I had just enough in me to get another mile but as partial miles didn't count, and I was beyond knackered, I called it quits. I had run eighty-four miles in twelve hours after having never run a step over 26.2 prior to that day. I received a few attaboys, a hand shake or two, and then I drove myself home. After eating and showering I crawled into bed and slept for no less than twelve straight hours. I only woke when the Judge I clerked for (himself also an avid runner) called to tell me I could come in a little late to work the next day, on Monday. I thanked him and more or less slept the rest of the day.

The feeling of telling all those who pledged a certain amount per mile what they owed me almost made up for how unbelievably wrecked my body was that next morning. If I had only known more about running, I would have never been so surprised at the things I would accomplish in the next few years. This race truly showed me was what possible when you simply go forth and try.

Race: Umstead 100

Typical Date: First Saturday in April

Distance: 100 miles

Location: Raleigh, NC

Why You Should Run It:

The Umstead 100-mile race is, if you can consider any 100-mile race easy, one of the easier ones to run. Or, more accurately, it enables runners who have difficulty finishing 100 miles in 24 hours, or just finishing 100 miles at all, the opportunity to do so when severe topography, heat, and getting lost are removed as major obstacles. While obviously weather can change for any race from year to year, the race correctly touts the fact that since it is held late March/early April, runners are normally treated to weather conducive to running well.

The course is a 12.5-mile loop which runners traverse eight different times, with a healthy 30-hour time limit to finish the distance. Run in the William B. Umstead State Park, the vast majority of the course is shaded and provides very clement weather conditions because of the tree coverage. The loop portion allows access to all the things a runner could need every few hours, which is wonderful when needs or desires change so often during the course of running for a day or more. With four water stops every loop, and your own supplies at the major rest area at the start/finish, it is a race which can be run almost entirely on the aid provided with no need for the runner to carry their own sustenance.

If you wish to have a crew or a runner follow you, you can after the fifth loop. But if you failed to utilize one, chances are you could pick up a random person to help you from an event which truly does have a family-feel to the entire proceeding. Also, unlike many ultras, because of the nature of the loops, you rarely feel alone or isolated.

The race has a 50-mile version occurring simultaneously as the 100 mile. An extremely underappreciated option is how, if you are not having a good day, you can choose to drop down from the 100 mile to the 50 mile. As I am big proponent of knowing when to stop and never needing to push through when it is unnecessary, I find this to be a huge bonus. Running ultras is hard enough without the crushing mental weight of thinking you ran 87 miles and got "nothing" for it. I've been there. If it isn't your day, call it quits and still receive a little solace as well.

My Experience:

I ran the Umstead 100 in 2010 one month before a much longer and more arduous event— my solo running of the 202-mile American Odyssey Relay. It was my second attempt at the 100 mile distance having DNFd the Old Dominion 100-mile race in 2007[191]. Going into the race I had been dealing with a variety of calf pains that I just could not shake. I would be fine once I started running but it would take me a good five miles before I didn't feel like I was tearing my calf off the bone. Nevertheless, I had grandiose plans entering this race. My training wasn't great but the weather was and I will take decent training and great weather over phenomenal training and awful weather any day of the week. I wasn't necessarily expecting to win the race but I thought perhaps if I had the day I knew I was capable of running, I could grab a podium spot.

Fortunately, any plans I had of wanting to win the race were more or less thrown out the window when I saw some of the runners there. Sure, anything can happen during a 100-miler, but when you are outclassed, you are just simply outclassed. The cream of the crop was Zach Gingerich, who I stood right behind in the bathroom line a mere five minutes before the race started. Wearing what can only be described as racing flats, I looked at him and thought: "I am going to get crushed today." With too many fast times to list, I knew about Zach's pedigree[192]. Also, no less than two other

---

[191] At mile 87, in second place, when I had given up at mile 75. Twelve miles on fumes was enough.

[192] He would win the Badwater Ultramarathon in Death Valley later that year, for example.

phenomenal runners were just milling around.

This knowledge actually made it easier to run my own race at my own pace. Nothing to win here, folks, move along. When the race started I found myself near the front which is where I should be given the pace I wanted to run. During this first loop I was just trying to find a rhythm. Even though I was not running much faster than my goal of 9:30 per mile, nothing felt quite right. Finally, after about six miles, the race began to fall into place. The first loop finished and the second loop began with me moving up in the standings and beginning to think those big thoughts again. I saw my buddy Andy Kumeda trucking along at an awesome clip. Andy and I had met for the first time at that first 100-miler I mentioned above where I had to call it a day. He churns out an impressive amount of these ultramarathons a year and I guess I should never be surprised to see him during a race.

Just a few miles into the third loop, everything started to go south. The energy was not there and I could tell it wasn't coming back. A good buddy of mine, Dean Schuster, was there to support some friends and was also giving me encouragement as well. He got me out of the chair to begin the fourth loop right around the time Zach was finishing his fourth. Wow. 50 miles in 6:18 with another 50 to go was amazing. I predicted to Dean that he was going to run 13:30. I was wrong. Zach ended up destroying the course record in 13:23.

A few miles into this fourth loop and I knew the day was done. I was finding it harder and harder to run on the flats and downhill portions, let alone contemplating doing so on an uphill. Now I just had to complete this loop and quit. Few things are harder than completing a course that you have already given up on but that was what I had to do. Perhaps I could have pressed on at a walk/jog pace, rallied and finished under 24 hour hours, snagging me a coveted belt buckle. But I had bigger fish to fry just 30 days away at the 202-miler, so I prudently called it a day.

It is always hard to quit earlier than expected than to continue to be "brave" and push on long past where you should have stopped.

However, I file this particular DNF under the category of "Do Nothing Foolish." It is almost always easier to push on through pain and exhaustion than it is to recognize you should stop for the longevity of your racing career. Or your life.

We live in world today where accolades are lauded upon those who post the most "vert" for their run or the bloodiest Instagram picture of their knees. Far too little praise is heaped upon those who know when it is wise to live to run another day. And there is always another race. Very few of us get paid to run. Even those who do get paid will rarely have an opportunity where a race is more important than their health. I am aware I am getting a little preachy here but this was one major lesson I learned from this race. Could I have pushed on, doing another four laps? Possibly. Was there any point to do so? No, not at all. Often races will give us harsh lessons which only become clear much later. Umstead gave me the lesson that sometimes it is ok to walk away.

Race: Hood to Coast

Typical Date: Last weekend before Labor Day

Distance: 199-mile relay

Location: Portland, OR

Why You Should Run It:

If you have run in virtually any relay of a long-distance nature you can more or less thank the Hood to Coast Relay for that fact it even exists. Beginning in 1982 with just eight teams, HTC has since become the gold standard in relays with over 1,000 teams running the event. So popular is this relay that for the last nineteen years it has filled its quota on opening day. You have to be faster registering than you do running just to get in.

The course runs approximately 200 miles (the course length varies due to small changes made by race organizers) from Timberline Lodge on the slopes of Mount Hood, the tallest peak in Oregon, through the Portland metropolitan area, and over to the beach town of Seaside on the Oregon Coast.

The relay was started by Portland architect Bob Foote, who was then president of Oregon Road Runners Club. The first relay in 1982 drew eight teams that ran 165 miles from Timberline to Kiwanda Beach near Pacific City, Oregon. The relay grew rapidly to over 400 teams by 1986. In 1989, the finish area was moved to Seaside where it remains today.

There may be races of this sort which traverse prettier parts of the country for longer periods of time, but to be part of the race which started all of them is to be a part of history.

My Experience:

My first experience with the race was as a spectator. Living in Portland, I found myself in town the weekend of the race. Being a big proponent of cheering on races that are around me if I am not running in them, I convinced my best friend to go down to a portion of the course which snaked its way just a few miles from my house. The best part was that we decided to do it around 1 a.m. which we thought would provide people with the biggest spark. We also found it scared the heck out of those who were running with headphones on playing music. I guess they weren't expecting a couple of running fans to be sitting on the course in the middle of the night. Word to the wise: stop running with music.

Two years later I was asked to join a team who had a late scratch because of an injury. Coincidentally, I was also just two weeks from a partial Achilles tear myself. However, I didn't want to miss this opportunity to take part and, promising to run conservatively, I joined the Fighting Squirrels. Relays are fantastic because of the intensity one can have during their own running and the silliness which can happen when they are not. The seriousness each runner takes with their own leg is balanced by how little others actually care about their teammates' performance during those very same legs. Didn't run your projected time? So? As long as you had fun and gave your best, the team is happy. Very few will berate their buddies who gave what they had that day. And if they do, I have a feeling those people are the ones who never get invited back.

Don't get me wrong: people take this race seriously, even if they are sandbagging how much they actually do care. This is because no one wants to be the weak link. Everyone wishes to be dependable. Need someone to run an extra mile (or four) because van traffic is so bad that vehicles take over two hours to go two miles? Well, pretty much every runner is happy to add to their total for the sake of the team. The team comes first.

In fact, the "team" becomes this amorphous entity which takes on a life and presence of its own. Even within the two separate groups of runners who barely interact, an ego and an id can rise and fall to balance one another out. One van is more stoic and anal; another is more wild and flying by the seat of its pants. Then that ingrained irrevocable identity can switch magically in the middle of the night from one group to the other. The "team" is finding its own yin and yang.

My team was comprised of 11 other great guys. It was an honor to be amongst them on this journey. In a little over 25 hours, we experienced lost runners, mixed up exchanges, nearly overturned Chevy Suburbans, tremendous gastrointestinal distress, and more inside jokes than normal people gather through months of being around each other.[193]

In the end, crossing the sand to the finish line was not a spiritual experience. But it wasn't far from one. I knew just one of my teammates before the race started. Now five of them are good friends and the six in the other van are, at the very least, close cousins.

The Squirrels put on a great show and ran well. More importantly we had a great time doing it. In addition, it sure was a bonus to know I picked up eleven more local running buddies. I can't wait to go searching for nuts with them.[194]

---

[193] "How many is a Brazilian?"
[194] Wait...that came out wrong.

The Cool Down

As I look over all the races in this book, I can immediately think of 52 more I would like to include. In fact, there are probably hundreds I hope to run before I hang up my running shoes for good which could be within these pages. However, I wanted to make sure that this book really grabbed the best of the best, and I could only put my stamp on them if I actually ran them. There are no less than twenty races I know I could recommend but as I haven't run them, that would be a bit disingenuous.

The racing world is becoming so diverse and full. I couldn't be happier to live in a time with such a vast array of races from which to choose. Gone are the days where running was the weird, fringe sport. Now, everyone is putting on a race. That means also that there are a lot of races which definitely do not make the cut. What I am hoping to do for you is not only reaffirm what you knew about some races, but let you know about others which may have been a mystery to you.

You most assuredly noticed how often I did not have the best racings days on races I have recommended in this book. If nothing else, that only solidifies why I think that even if you happen to have a similarly bad day, you too will enjoy the race nonetheless. Some of my fastest races ever have been on very-well put together events by wonderful people. They just didn't necessarily stand out above others as an event I truly feel everyone should want to run.

Once I ran the Marine Corps Marathon, went home, showered, and came back to the finish. Some runners were talking about a huge bottleneck on the Metro, how the Marines were swamped with runners coming in, and a few other things that I, when I finished 117th, had not experienced. That race drove it into my head how two people, running the same race, on the same day, can truly experience completely separate races. So while my own experiences were paramount to inclusion in this book, every race here also took into account the tales I read from others at various points along the course. It also helped to remind me that no race is perfect. There will be snafus. There will be hiccups. We must remember how much goes into all races, even those which aren't necessarily all that special. More often than not, races are put on by other runners, just hoping to provide their brethren with a great running day.

Rest assured that as I continue to race, I will chronicle all those events in my notes and in my mind. I hope to provide you with another list of races not only in North America but abroad as well. Until I am able to do so, I think you will find these races contained within this book will leave you with ample challenges, in wonderful locales, for which you can whet the tongues of your running shoes.

See you at the finish line!

Special Thanks to these Kickstarter Backers

John Mehall, Patricia Reynolds Vanderwest, Mike Durhamm, Jill Crawford, Manfred Schmidt, Scott Nash, Damaris Rosich-Schwartz, Terry Hoebelheinrich, Giovanny León, Heather Alvarado Rine, Lane Blake, Jenny Rutherford, Michael Kelly, Greg Johnson, Casey Anthony, Heather Vachon, Anthony Portera, Mark McInerney, Ed Childress, Monique Savits, Matt Borland, Emmanuel Moustakakis, Carl Olson, Connie Brown, Robert Bailey, Peter Pressman, Michelle Hylton, Tammy Massie, Dave McGillivray, Mary Beth Koeth, Laura Lee Patterson, Steve Pheby, Kevin Baumgartner, Maurice Lee III, Danny Fleener, John Roman, Dale Johnston, Dean Jaeger, Ross Kinney, Teri Poulton, Sonia Ho, Kim Harris, Heather Kvasnak, Gary Acosta, Barb Rauschenberg, Lindsay Jameson.